Brain Control

Also by David Linden

THE BIOLOGY OF PSYCHOLOGICAL DISORDERS

Brain Control

Developments in Therapy and Implications for Society

David Linden
Cardiff University Schools of Medicine and Psychology, UK

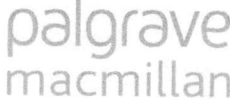

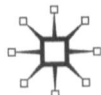
First published 2014 by
PALGRAVE MACMILLAN

Palgrave Macmillan in the UK is an imprint of Macmillan Publishers Limited, registered in England, company number 785998, of Houndmills, Basingstoke, Hampshire RG21 6XS.

Palgrave Macmillan in the US is a division of St Martin's Press LLC, 175 Fifth Avenue, New York, NY 10010.

Palgrave Macmillan is the global academic imprint of the above companies and has companies and representatives throughout the world.

Palgrave® and Macmillan® are registered trademarks in the United States, the United Kingdom, Europe and other countries

ISBN: 978–1–137–33532–6

This book is printed on paper suitable for recycling and made from fully managed and sustained forest sources. Logging, pulping and manufacturing processes are expected to conform to the environmental regulations of the country of origin.

A catalogue record for this book is available from the British Library.

Library of Congress Cataloging-in-Publication Data

Linden, David, 1968–
    Brain control : developments in therapy and implications for society / David Linden.
        pages cm
        ISBN 978–1–137–33532–6 (hardback)
    1. Brain stimulation. 2. Biofeedback training. 3. Psychosurgery. 4. Brain – Localization of functions. 5. Neurosciences – Moral and ethical aspects. 6. Neurosciences – Social aspects. I. Title.

QP388.L56 2014
612.8′22—dc23   2014024398

Transferred to Digital Printing in 2014

Contents

List of Figures

Acknowledgements

I am grateful to Professor David Healy for invaluable advice on the history of physical treatments in psychiatry, to Professor Dieter Müller for information about the German hypothalamotomy programme, to Professor Bruno Millet for information about psychiatric Deep Brain Stimulation and to Professors Rainer Goebel and Christoph Klein for frequent discussions about neurofeedback. My wife, Dr Stefanie Linden, taught me how to turn the complex material into an engaging story. My collaborators on the neurofeedback programme at Cardiff University, Dr Leena Subramanian, Isabelle Habes, Dr Niklas Ihssen and Dr Moses Sokunbi, kindly provided illustrations and case histories for Chapter 3. I am also very grateful to Professor Volker Arnd Coenen for providing Figure 2.5. Caroline Delgado, the widow and longstanding collaborator of Dr Jose Delgado, kindly gave permission to reproduce material from his book and provided a fascinating vignette of her late husband's research. None of these colleagues can be presumed to endorse the content of this book and all errors are the sole responsibility of the author.

Figure 1.4 has been reprinted from Linden DE, Prvulovic D, Formisano E, et al, "The functional neuroanatomy of target detection: an fMRI study of visual and auditory oddball tasks", *Cereb Cortex*, 1999, 9(8): 815–823, by permission of Oxford University Press.

Figure 2.6 has been reprinted from Rodriguez-Oroz MC, Jahanshahi M, Krack P, et al, "Initial clinical manifestations of Parkinson's disease: features and pathophysiological mechanisms", *Lancet Neurol*, 2009, 8(12): 1128–1139, with permission from Elsevier.

Figure 3.4 has been reprinted from Esmail S, Linden D, "Emotion regulation networks and neurofeedback in depression", *Cognitive Sciences*, 2011, 6(2), with permission from Nova Science Publishers, Inc.

Figure 3.5 printed with the permission of Professor Roger Whitaker.

Introduction

The technology for brain stimulation and brain reading has developed rapidly over the last two decades. Deep Brain Stimulation (DBS) is now well established as a treatment for movement disorders while psychiatric applications are also emerging. Brain Computer Interfaces (BCIs) enable communication and control in laboratory settings and first applications on patients with complete paralysis are under way. Finally, neurofeedback, which enables patients to self-regulate their own brain activity, is being explored as a new treatment for neuropsychiatric disorders that combines elements from traditional physical and psychological therapies.

The techniques for brain control and self-control share a common history, which reaches back to the early electrical stimulation studies of the 19th century. It is a story not only of failure and controversy but also of fascinating innovation and therapeutic success. Brain control is also an area of increasing clinical and social importance. Over 60,000 patients with Parkinson's disease have been treated with DBS, and programmes to roll out this technique for patients with depression, one of the major epidemics of our time, are gaining momentum. BCIs for communication and control could potentially revolutionise the care of hundreds of thousands of patients with spinal cord and brain injuries. At the same time, there are considerable fears that techniques for brain reading and control could violate privacy and be used to manipulate people's minds.

This book describes the attempts over the last 150 years to influence and change brain and behaviour through external and internal stimulation, surgical operations and training. It covers animal experiments, such as the reprogramming of flight responses in chickens, and studies in human patients, such as those leading to the successful treatment of

1

movement disorders with DBS. We will encounter patients who have benefited from the insertion of electrodes into their brains or from surgery to modify behaviour, and patients who have developed disabling side effects. This book also explains how we can read the brain of patients who cannot communicate in other ways and how this information can be used to give them back some control over their lives through brain-computer interfaces. The author was motivated to write this book by his own experience in developing "neurofeedback" protocols for giving patients with mental disorders or brain degeneration control over their own brains. We will look at the development of these new treatments and explore whether they can make a real contribution to improving the lives of the growing number of people with depression or Parkinson's disease.

"Brain control" thus not only embraces situations in which doctors take control of a patient's brain, but also techniques that enable patients themselves to gain control over their brains. Such brain training need not be confined to the treatment of patients with psychiatric or neurological disorders but could also be used to change aspects of one's personality or improve cognitive functions. These non-therapeutic applications of brain enhancement pose pressing ethical issues, and the increasing availability of devices that allow people to train their own brains makes them even more topical. In the last section of the book we will therefore review the current regulation of brain enhancement and suggest ways in which society can and should utilise techniques for brain control.

1
Putting the Brain in Control: From Brain Reading to Brain Communication

1.1 Locked-in

When Jean-Dominique Bauby, a successful French journalist and editor of the fashion magazine *Elle*, suffered a stroke in 1995 at the age of 43 his life changed completely. The stroke had affected his brainstem and when he awoke from three weeks in a coma he found himself unable to talk or move his limbs. He could only communicate through opening or closing his eyes to indicate yes or no responses. However, he was able to process information from the outside world through his sensory channels, to think, feel, evoke old memories and form new ones. We know this because, true to his profession, he went on to dictate a book, *Le Scaphandre et le Papillon* (*The Diving Bell and the Butterfly*), with the help of a speech therapist who had devised a system whereby he could form words by picking letters from visually presented streams using his eye blink responses. His book, which was also adapted into a movie, became a bestseller immediately after its release in March 1997, but Bauby died a few days after publication. Shortly before his death from pneumonia he had set up an association for those suffering from the same condition, the *Association du Locked-in Syndrome*.

The term locked-in syndrome describes a state when the brain is disconnected from the body and thus is locked into the skull. It can occur after lesions of the upper brainstem, the part that connects the command areas in the cerebral hemispheres with the rest of the body (except for some of the sensory channels; which explains why he could still see, hear and smell). Such lesions can be caused suddenly by a stroke or surreptitiously by motor neuron disease (MND) (also called amyotrophic lateral sclerosis (ALS)), a progressive degeneration of the motor neurons of the brain and spinal cord. Because the higher areas of the

3

brain, the parts supporting consciousness, are generally not affected, patients are fully alert and aware of the outside world. Yet, because these higher areas of the brain are disconnected from the motor pathways that convey commands to the periphery of the body, patients have almost no control over their muscles and thus cannot walk, talk or interact with their environment in any other way, except by gaze or blink movements. These movements are only spared because their control involves nerves that leave the brain at very high levels, above those affected by the lesion, in a structure called the midbrain.

However, patients with lesions that are located even higher up in the brain may ultimately become completely paralysed and unable to engage in any way with their environment. All their movements will be reflexive and not under voluntary control. For these patients, reading questions and answers directly from their brain would be the only way to communicate. Some highly publicised efforts have evolved around the development of devices to enable the famous Cambridge physicist Professor Stephen Hawking, a longstanding MND sufferer, to communicate should he ever lose control over his facial muscles, which he is currently using to operate a computer. Although this may have sounded like science fiction just decades ago, modern brain recording techniques and fast computers now make this a real possibility.

1.2   Motor control: from brain to muscle

All our movements are produced by muscle contractions, which occur when the filaments of the two proteins actin and myosin slide against each other. The biochemical processes that result in these protein movements are triggered by the release of charged calcium particles from stores within the muscle cells. This release of calcium is triggered in turn by electrical changes in the cell that arise from its connection with a nerve at the, so-called, motor endplate (Figure 1.1). At the endplate an incoming electrical impulse is converted into a chemical signal, the release of the neurotransmitter acetylcholine, which docks onto specific receptors on the muscle cell membrane. Neurotransmitters are chemicals released by neurons that mediate the communication with other cells. Through binding to its receptor, acetylcholine opens a pore in the membrane, through which ions, small charged particles, can travel into the muscle cell and excite it electrically.

The nerve cell that connects with the muscle at the endplate commonly has its cell body in the spinal cord (Figure 1.1). Nerve cells, or neurons, have a cell body that contains the DNA (deoxyribonucleic acid), the repository of genetic information in its nucleus, and generally

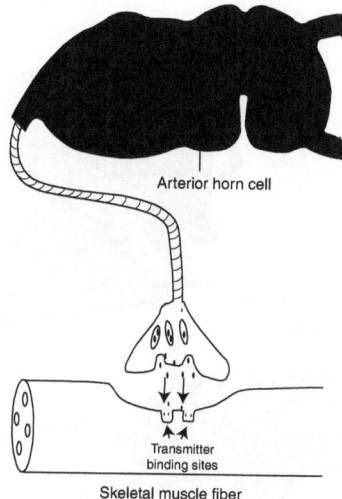

Figure 1.1   Neural control of muscle activity

Note: The axons of motor neurons in the anterior horn of the spinal connect with skeletal muscle fibres to form a motor unit. The motor neuron releases a transmitter substance that leads to changes in the electrical property of the muscle fibre and can induce it to contract. Not drawn to scale.

one main output cable, the axon, which can be several metres long in large animals. It receives its input through a system of dendrites, which can contain hundreds or even thousands of little branches. On each of these branches there can be connections (called synapses) from other neurons. A neuron can thus be connected to thousands of other neurons, which is the basis for the huge complexity of the brain. The motor nerve cell in the spinal cord, also called lower motor neuron, receives input from an upper motor neuron in the motor control area of the brain, the primary motor cortex (Figure 1.2). One important feature of the motor pathways from the brain to the spinal cord is that they cross from one side to the other – thus movements of the right arm or leg are under the control of the left motor cortex and vice versa.

The initiation of a movement also involves other brain areas which are involved in motor preparation, planning and control, but a simple movement, such as the twitching of the right thumb, can be generated just by a stimulation of the appropriate area of primary motor cortex. Because the axons from upper to lower motor neurons cross over at the level of the lower brainstem, the control centre for the right hand is in the left motor cortex. And it is not even necessary to undergo brain

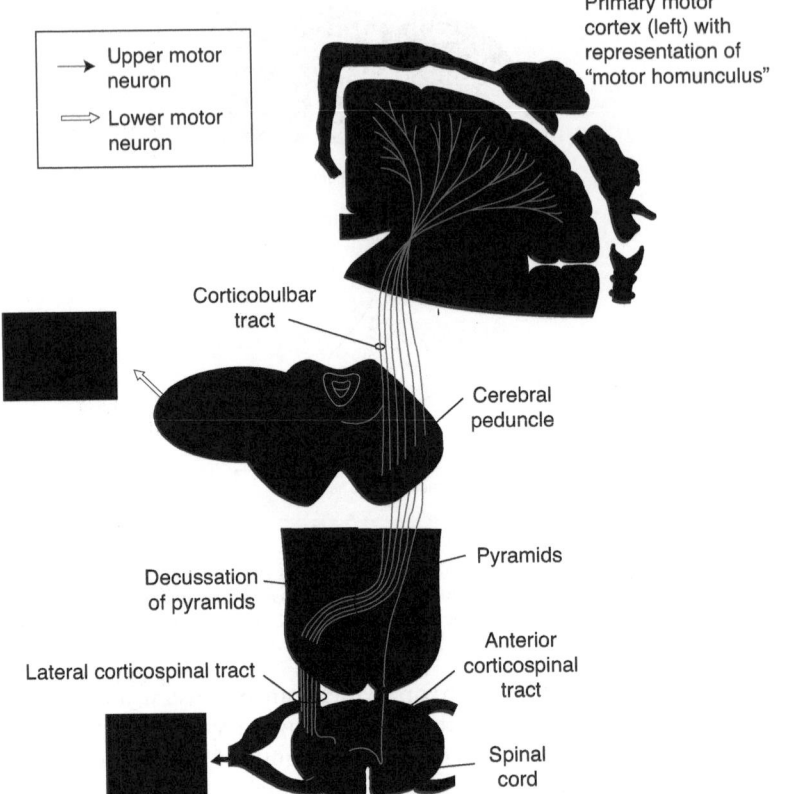

Figure 1.2   The cortico-spinal motor pathways

Note: The main motor pathway originates in the primary motor cortex of the frontal lobe of the brain, where motor neurons are arranged according to the body part to which they project ("somatotopy", graphically depicted through the homunculus). Projections to muscles of the face and neck leave at the level of the brainstem through the motor portions of the cranial nerves. Projections to the limbs and trunk cross to the other side and travel down the spinal cord. For their further connection with skeletal muscles see Figure 1.1.

surgery to create such a stimulation. Non-invasive devices that deliver electromagnetic impulses through the intact skull (transcranially) are powerful enough to induce such movements, even if the stimulated person tries to prevent it. This method is called Transcranial Magnetic Stimulation (TMS). Brain stimulation thus allows us to map out functional areas and if we have the option of stimulating the brain during operations directly we can obtain very detailed maps, for example the homunculus of motor representations in the primary motor cortex (Figure 1.2). This area contains the upper motor neurons responsible for movement of the whole body apart from the eyes, which have a separate motor region called the frontal eye fields, a few centimetres in front of the primary motor cortex.

If the connections between the upper and lower motor neurons are severed, one can still form the intention to execute a movement, but the commands then cannot arrive at the appropriate muscles. If both motor tracts are cut through a lesion or otherwise destroyed (e.g. through a bleed or tumour) in the uppermost parts of the spinal cord in the neck the person will be unable to move their arms or legs. They will be tetra-plegic (Greek: *tetra* – four; *plegia* – paralysis), meaning that they cannot move any of their four limbs. In these patients TMS, or even direct cortical stimulation during surgery, cannot evoke limb movements because, although the motor cortex is intact, it is no longer connected with the periphery.

If the lesion is located even higher in the brain it will, in addition, affect the pathways to the cranial nerves that control the muscles of the face and eye and thus make it impossible for the patient to articulate speech or to swallow, as in the cases of advanced MND or brainstem stroke. Only the cranial nerves that leave the brain above the level of the lesion will receive input from the motor control areas. With lesions high up in the midbrain the only nerves that are still connected to the higher motor areas may be the branches for blinking and vertical eye movements, as in the case of Jean-Dominique Bauby. The patient, or more precisely the brain, is thus almost completely locked-in, and if they go on to lose the ability to blink and move their eyes they would not have any way of expressing themselves.

How then can modern technology help locked-in patients link with the outside world? The basic idea is simple; if we can read patients' thoughts and intentions from the intact, higher areas of their brains we might be able to communicate with them directly in the language of the brain rather than through the defective speech apparatus. The devil, though, is in the mathematical and physiological detail. At present it is not possible to read information about individual thoughts through the intact skull, and even with invasive recordings it takes many years of training for patients to convert their intentions into relatively simple motor commands (see Section 1.9). However, patients can be trained to give yes/no responses through changes in their brain activity, similar to the blinking code used by Jean-Dominique Bauby. The technique behind this simplest form of brain reading is called electroencephalography (EEG).

1.3   The electric brain

Electrical potentials in the brain can be picked up through the intact skull by EEG. The discovery and initial development of this technique was the achievement of German psychiatrist Hans Berger (1873–1941).[1] Berger published his first paper on this method in 1929. What was amazing, and hitherto unknown, was the regularity of the waves of neural activity that could be picked up from the human brain during both the wake state and in sleep. The main oscillation had a frequency between 8 Hertz (Hz) and 12 Hz (8–12 peaks per second) and was called alpha rhythm by Berger. Its exact origins in the brain are still unknown but Berger knew that it must be some sort of resting or default activity of the wake brain because he could suppress it by asking his subjects to engage in effortful mental activity, for example mental arithmetic. Such manipulation brought about faster, smaller waves, which he called beta rhythm. Conversely, when subjects dozed off their EEG became slower. Heated debates on the functional significance of EEG rhythms arose immediately after Berger published his findings, for example between him and the leading British neurophysiologist Edgar (later Lord) Adrian, 1932 Nobel laureate. Adrian and his colleague Bryan Matthews conducted a series of experiments which ruled out that the EEG rhythms were artefacts arising outside the brain, for example from eye movement, supporting Berger's view that the EEG reflected nerve activity in the brain. Yet they also contradicted Berger's view that the alpha rhythm, called Berger rhythm by Adrian in honour of its discoverer, was generated throughout the brain and tried to localise its origin in the occipital areas at the back of the brain, the site of the visual cortex. Because opening the eyes suppresses the Berger rhythm (Figure 1.3), in the same way as effortful mental activity did, they concluded that this

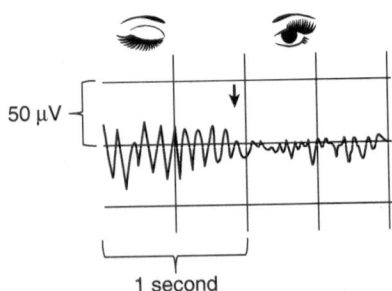

Figure 1.3 EEG trace with eyes closed (showing the alpha, or Berger, rhythm) and opened (showing the suppression of the rhythm)

rhythm represented the synchronous oscillation of the visual cortex at rest, which was disrupted by visual stimulation.[2]

Adrian and Matthews also conducted the first neurofeedback experiment (although they did not use this term), whereby they converted the amplitude of EEG activity into sound signals and monitored the EEG changes produced by opening and closing the eyes:

> Again some of the evidence on the effect of opening the eyes in the dark was made by one of us listening to the rhythm from his head in a loud speaker. This made it possible to correlate the impression of not looking or looking with the presence or absence of the rhythm. In this case, as when the eyes are opened in daylight, the subject can hear that the rhythm ceases.[2]

Over many decades EEG was the main tool for registering brain activity non-invasively in humans. Because EEG has a very high temporal resolution and can track the activation of neural networks at a millisecond scale researchers developed techniques that allowed them to couple EEG recordings with the presentation of specific stimuli and then trace the sequence of activation across the brain. Such evoked potential studies have been conducted with all types of sensory stimulus. For example, after the presentation of a picture one can record the first evoked potential over the visual cortex after 70 ms–100 ms, followed by waves that correspond to specific stimulus properties or to the cognitive task of the participant. One particularly well-studied brain wave is the P300, a positive wave starting about 300 ms after the presentation of a stimulus, which indexes attention and working memory (Figure 1.4). It is most strongly evoked by, so-called, oddball protocols, where a regular sequence of stimuli is disrupted by a rare stimulus, the oddball. For example if rare high tones are interspersed in sequences of low tones, the high tones will evoke a P300. Conversely, if the low tones are rare and the high tones common, the low tones will evoke the P300. This wave can even be evoked by the omission of an expected stimulus. It thus indexes expectancy, which is the product of attention and memory, rather than any specific attributes of the stimulus. In fact, it can be evoked in relatively similar fashion by pictures, sounds or tactile stimuli.

The P300 therefore allows researchers to gain some insight into the mental state of a person, for example by determining whether a particular stimulus was expected or not. This wave is of interest for brain communication devices because, to some extent, it is under voluntary control. If a locked-in patient can be trained to produce a P300 whenever he or she

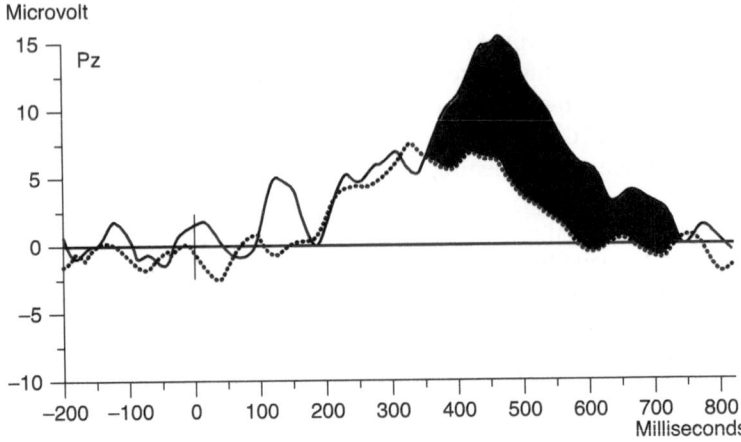

Figure 1.4   Example of the P300 wave evoked by rare stimuli (filled line), but not frequent stimuli (dotted line) in a visual oddball paradigm

Note: The EEG trace was recorded at electrode Pz, which describes a location centrally above the parietal lobe. Adapted from Linden, Prvulovic, Formisano, Völlinger, Zanella, Goebel and Dierks 1999[3] with kind permission of Oxford University Press.

sees the letter that comes next in the word that they are trying to form, even patients without the capacity to move their eyes or blink could ultimately dictate letters, or even books like Jean-Dominique Bauby. We will see that such a P300 speller is indeed one of the potential brain computer interfaces being developed for brain communication with paralysed patients.

Another important way of categorising EEG activity uses the main frequency of its oscillatory rhythm. The frequency bands below Berger's alpha rhythm (8 Hz–12 Hz) are called theta (3.5 Hz–8 Hz) and delta (below 3.5 Hz) bands. They are dominant during deep sleep. Conversely, during cognitive activation the EEG can go into higher frequency oscillations, in the beta (12 Hz–30 Hz) or gamma (30 Hz–100 Hz) bands,[4] although the higher range of this activity is of low intensity and can only be extracted by computer analysis rather than be appreciated with the naked eye (Figure 1.5). Such computer analysis of the frequency spectrum can also be used to feed the relative strength of these frequency bands back to a person in real-time and train them to change this pattern through neurofeedback (NF). One example is the study of young musicians who were trained to increase their theta rhythm to improve performance (see Section 3.2).

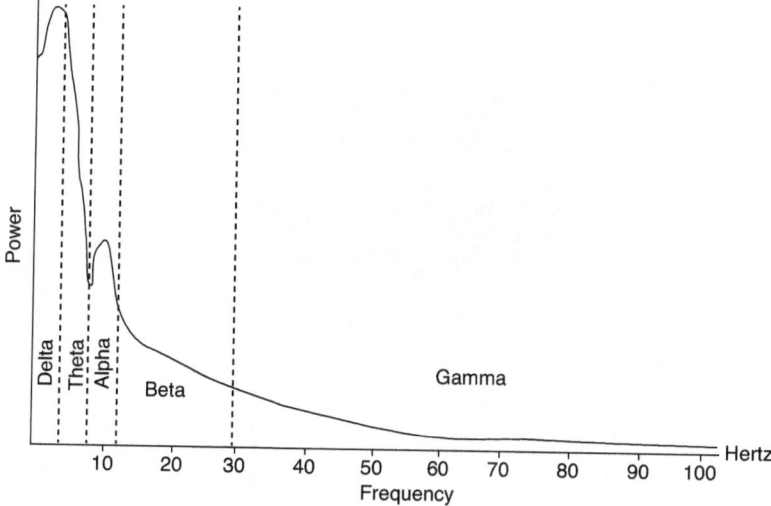

Figure 1.5   The frequency bands of the EEG

Note: The contribution of different frequency bands to the EEG at rest. The contribution to the overall electrical activity is inversely related to the frequency, with the exception of a peak in the alpha range. Cognitive activity can be associated with further peaks in the higher (beta, gamma) frequency ranges.

1.4   The biggest network in the universe

Even a high resolution EEG cap with 256 electrodes only captures the complexity of the brain in very crude ways. The human brain contains about 80 billion (1 billion = 1,000,000,000) neurons, more than the estimated number of stars in the universe. About 20% of the neurons are located in the cerebral hemispheres, forming a 2 mm–4 mm thick sheet called the cerebral cortex. The cerebral hemispheres are conventionally divided into four lobes, the frontal lobe at the front, the parietal lobe in the middle, the occipital lobe at the back and the temporal lobe at the side (Figure 1.6). About 80% of our neurons are located in an area called the cerebellum, which is chiefly concerned with fine tuning of movements and balance, where the neurons are particularly densely packed. The rest of the brain, including the basal ganglia and the brainstem, accounts for less than 1% of brain neurons.

A degeneration of even a relatively small number of neurons in these regions can lead to major clinical consequences. For example, there are only about 600,000 neurons that produce the neurotransmitter dopamine

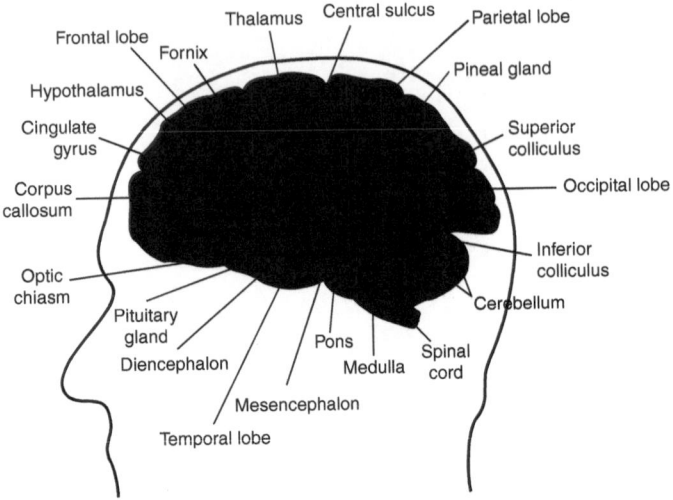

Figure 1.6 Overview of brain areas. From Linden[5] with kind permission of Palgrave Macmillan

Note: This schematic section through the midline (cuts in this direction are called 'sagittal views') shows many of the brain areas discussed in this book..

in the human brain. Although this number is tiny when compared to the overall 80 billion, the degeneration of these neurons in the midbrain leads to the severe impairment of motor function that is seen in Parkinson's disease.

With each neuron able to form thousands of connections with other neurons through its branching dendrites, the potential number of paths through which information can be passed between neurons is in the trillions, although the actual number is unknown and may vary greatly between individuals (whereas there is likely to be much less variability between healthy individuals in the overall number of neurons). Until recently it was assumed that humans do not grow any new neurons after birth, although this may be too pessimistic. There is now good evidence for new neurons being formed in the adult hippocampus,[6] a key region for learning and memory. However, the main mechanism for the huge amount of learning that goes on from birth to adulthood and across the lifespan seems to be the formation of new connections between neurons, rather than the generation of new neurons.

The main structural basis for connectivity between neurons is the contact (synapse) between two neurons. This synapse is formed by the terminal membrane of a branch of the axon of the first neuron and the cell membrane of the second. It is outside the scope of this book to go into much more detail on the structure and physiology of the synapse and neuronal connections, but this has been described in many introductory textbooks of neuroscience.[5]

The neurons do not touch directly but leave a space of a few hundred nanometres between them (1 nanometre = 1 billionth of a meter), which is called the synaptic cleft. The principle of communication between neurons is similar to that between neuron and muscle introduced in Section 1.2. An incoming electrical signal travelling down the axon of the first neuron leads to the release of a chemical, the neurotransmitter, which then docks onto receptors on the second neuron and changes its chemical and electrical properties. In this way electrical information is converted into chemical information and back into electrical information. If the electrical excitation of the second neuron surpasses a certain threshold it generates an impulse it its own axon, called action potential, which can in turn excite further neurons in the network. If its excitation remains below a certain threshold the neuron will remain silent. Any single neuron can be thus conceived of as an input–output machine, which receives chemical and/or electrical signals and converts them into an output in an all-or-nothing fashion.

If the brain only consisted of excitatory loops of the sort just described it would be in constant uncontrolled activity and soon be depleted of its energy reserves. Synapses act like miniature batteries, and batteries of any size need energy. In the case of neuronal batteries the energy is supplied by a molecule called ATP (adenosine triphosphate), whose production is fuelled by the glucose that we derive from our nutrition. Balance and control of neural activity is achieved through the interplay between excitatory and inhibitory neurons. Inhibitory neurons release neurotransmitters that make a neuron less excitable. The simplest example of such an excitatory/inhibitory system is the reflex arc described in Figure 1.7. When we extend our leg the opposing muscles responsible for bending the leg need to be inhibited in order to avoid a cramp. Although this is an example from the peripheral nervous system (the part downstream from the spinal cord), similar mechanisms of inhibitory control operate throughout the central nervous system (the brain and spinal cord) as well.

1.5 Conditioning the brain

Reflexive, automatic actions and their neural mechanisms were the core interest of the leading neurophysiologists of the late 19th and early 20th centuries. Sir Charles Sherrington (1857–1952), for example, who shared the Nobel Prize with Adrian in 1932, spent a long and extremely fruitful

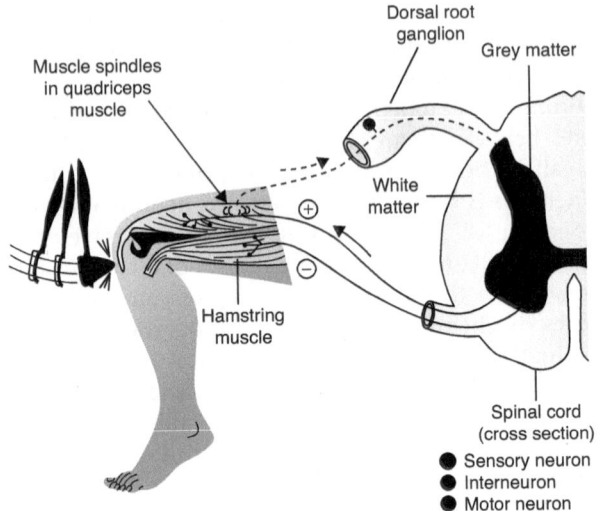

Figure 1.7   The reflex arc of the knee jerk illustrates basic principles of excitatory and inhibitory neuronal activity

Note: A tap on the tendon of the quadriceps muscle below the patella stretches the muscle, which activates muscle spindles. These are connected to sensory nerves (broken lines) that project through the dorsal root onto motor neurons in the anterior horn (black) and inhibitory interneurons (grey). They activate the innervation of their own muscle, which then contracts to counteract the stretch, resulting in the knee jerk. At the same time, the motor neurons for the antagonist (hamstring muscle) are inhibited by the activated interneurons. From Linden[5] with kind permission of Palgrave Macmillan.

scientific life studying the nerve connections that gave rise to the knee jerk and other important reflexes. However, at the same time a field of research was emerging that was to show that many of these physiological reflexes were not completely hard-wired and immutable but could be modified or even produced by classical or instrumental conditioning.

The Russian physician Ivan Petrovitch Pavlov (1849–1936) demonstrated that vegetative reflexes under the control of the autonomic nervous system could be conditioned. The American psychologists Edward Lee Thorndike (1874–1949), John Broadus Watson (1878–1958) and Burrhus Frederic Skinner (1904–1990), pioneers of animal behaviour research, suggested that almost any overt behaviour could be changed by reinforcement. Was this true also for physiological responses? Could animals be trained to change their heart rate in the same way they could be trained to press a lever or find the way out of a puzzle box?

Let us briefly consider how this might work. If animals learn from the consequences of their actions, as Thorndike had posited in his fundamental Law of Effect, they have to receive some feedback on their actions. In standard operant conditioning this would be a reward signalling to them that they had opened the right box, pressed the right lever, or whatever the possible actions in the laboratory setup were. If one wanted to train an animal to regulate a physiological response rather than to make a specific movement one would have to replace the contingency "lever press then food" with "reduce heart rate then food". Animals should then learn to reduce their heart rate in much the same way as they learnt to press a lever. The pulse meter could signal to the animal to engage in this task again in the same way as being put into a Skinner box or seeing a green light signals to the animal to start the lever pressing task. However, the analogy is not quite as straightforward. Whereas pressing a lever is well within the natural repertoire of behaviours of a rat – in fact they start manipulating levers and other objects in the cage even if no reward is provided at all – actively changing its heart rate is not. This will make the gradual shaping of the desired behaviours and activities more difficult. Also, animals receive feedback about their movements from at least two sources. One is the, so-called, efference copy that is sent from the motor centres to the sensory centres in order to allow them to distinguish between active and passive movements; the other are the peripheral signals on the position of the relevant limb, which come from position sensors in the limbs themselves (the so-called proprioceptive system), through visual observation of the limb or through other sensory channels. Yet no such direct information is available about most physiological signals, perhaps with the exception of salivation, which we can feel on our skin. Changes in heart rate, blood pressure or skin conductance, when they are subtle, are not obvious to our senses. For feedback training the experimenter thus needs to transform them into a sensory signal, for example playing a tone for every heartbeat. Such direct, on-line information about physiological signals is central to procedures that come under the heading of biofeedback.

In the 1950s and 1960s neuroscientists started research programmes both on classical and operant conditioning of neural activity. Physiologists Robert Doty and Corneliu Giurgea conducted classical conditioning with electrical stimulation in two different areas of the brains of dogs and monkeys. They used electrical activation of an area that produced a distinctive motor response, for example bending of a foreleg, as the unconditioned stimulus (US). At the same time they applied electrical pulses to another brain area, which in isolation did not elicit any response. This was the conditioned stimulus (CS), and after only a few days of training, the CS alone could evoke the same motor response as the US. These results challenged the idea that the brain of adult animals (including humans) is essentially hard-wired for certain functions and suggests that relatively brief, but specific, training can change the functions of a brain area, even to the extent that it produces completely different movements from before.[7] Elegant experiments by Andrew Jackson, Jaideep Mavoori and Eberhard Fetz at the University of Washington in Seattle over forty years later confirmed that the motor systems of the brain are amazingly plastic. They implanted a recording electrode into one part of the motor cortex (site 1) of a monkey and connected it to a stimulation electrode implanted into another part of motor cortex (site 2) with a neurochip, which, whenever it picked up a signal from site 1, stimulated site 2 (within a few milliseconds, this close temporal pairing is crucial), evoking the motor response produced by activation of site 2. Both sites produced different movements of the contralateral wrist. After the neurons in site 1 had been conditioned with this protocol for a few days, the wrist torque generated by activation of site 1 alone deviated the wrist from its original direction and moved it towards the direction generated when site 2 was stimulated directly.[8]

One interpretation is that the process of consistently pairing activation of two areas (whether through paired stimulation as in Doty and Giurgea's experiments or whether through an artificial electrical connection as in Jackson and Fetz's experiments) leads to new connections between these two areas. Such a mechanism for neuroplasticity and learning where "neurons that fire together wire together" had originally been postulated by the Canadian psychologist Donald Hebb in his 1949 book *The Organization of Behavior*:

> When an axon of cell A is near enough to excite a cell B and repeatedly or persistently takes part in firing it, some growth process or metabolic change takes place in one or both cells such that A's efficiency, as one of the cells firing B, is increased.[9]

In parallel with Doty and Giurgea's work on the classical conditioning of neural activity researchers also started operant training of neural responses. Hebb's pupil James Olds trained animals to up- or downregulate the activity of single nerve cells. He rewarded the desired neural responses with electrical stimulation of the medial forebrain bundle, which he established to be a very potent reward for rodents, as we will see in Section 2.3. Olds thus conducted the first neurofeedback studies in animals. He observed relatively fast neural learning in the hippocampus and other parts of the limbic system.[10] In the 1960s, Eberhard Fetz trained monkeys to control the activity of single neurons in the motor command centres.[11] Starting from the work by Olds and Fetz in the 1950s and 1960s, numerous studies have subsequently confirmed that, in non-paralysed animals, neurofeedback works. Rats could even be trained to regulate their brain activity in one or other direction to get a food or drink reward, depending on whether they were hungry or thirsty.[12] However, these experiments suffered from a potentially crucial confound: animals may have merely learnt certain subtle movement patterns that produced the desired neural effects – similar to Adrian's rather crude use of eyelid movement to influence the Berger rhythm. This possibility could only be ruled out by paralysing the animal, which was the theme of a series of studies conducted by American psychologist Neal Elgar Miller over several decades.

The pioneers of operant conditioning of physiological responses in the 1950s and 1960s faced an uphill struggle because the standard view was that only voluntary motor acts could be brought under operant control, whereas autonomic responses – as implied by the term – could only be modified by classical conditioning. In 1961 the leading American psychologist Gregory Adams Kimble, editing the standard textbook of learning theory, had stated that,

> for autonomically mediated behavior, the evidence points unequivocally to the conclusion that such responses can be modified by classical, but not instrumental, training methods.[13]

Miller, working first at Yale and later at Rockefeller University in New York City was unperturbed. Miller was an authority on animal learning and had a longstanding interest in links between learning theory and psychotherapy. In addition to his background in animal behaviour and physiology, he had trained in psychoanalysis in Vienna in the 1930s and had published a book on *Personality and Psychotherapy* in 1950. One major problem he faced in his quest to demonstrate operant conditioning of physiological responses was that most physiological changes can be produced by voluntary movements. For example, we can increase our heart rate simply by walking faster, or influence blood pressure by the tension and relaxation of muscles. This last relationship had already been studied by the Chicago-born physician Edmund Jacobson in the 1930s and served as the foundation of his technique of progressive muscle relaxation. Would it be possible to demonstrate a control over physiological responses that is not mediated simply by operant conditioning of skeletal muscle actions? There were encouraging, yet controversial, observations from the field of classical conditioning. Russian physiologists had chemically blocked the salivary glands of dogs while they were conducting Pavlov's experiments. The dog thus never actually produced any saliva during the conditioning procedure. Yet, when the chemical block was removed, the dog salivated to the sound and thus showed the normal conditioned response. Similarly, fear responses could be conditioned in animals paralysed with curare, and thus without any motor responses during the learning procedure. When the effect of the curare wore off, the animals still showed the expected avoidant behaviour to the conditioned stimulus.[14] This implied that peripheral physiological changes during conditioning were not required and that all the relevant processes occurred in the central nervous system. In order to obtain analogous effects with operant conditioning Miller had to ensure that the animals had no control over their skeletal muscles and therefore paralysed them with curare. Incidentally, curare and its derivatives only block neural signalling to the skeletal muscles and not to the heart and other visceral organs, which means that autonomic physiological responses, such as heart rate changes, can still be observed. However, curarised animals cannot swallow, and thus Miller could not use normal food or drink rewards and had to resort to direct stimulation of the brain's reward centres, similar to those pioneered by Olds in the 1950s. With this procedure he managed to train rats, over several weeks, to increase or decrease their heart rate by 20% upon specific signals. Even more stunningly, animals also learnt to regulate bowel and kidney function, such as the amount of urine they produced. When Miller had managed to train rats to regulate the blood supply to their ears he expressed his surprise with a candour rarely encountered in current scientific papers:

> We were somewhat surprised and greatly delighted to find that this experiment actually worked.[15]

Miller and his colleagues even went on to train brain activity. He moved from biofeedback to neurofeedback, where animals are rewarded not for changing a peripheral physiological response such as heart rate or salivation, but for showing an alteration in brain activity as measured on, for instance, the EEG. They rewarded cats, again with electrical stimulation of the MFB, for increasing or lowering the amplitude of brain waves by about 30%, which they recorded with electrodes on the brain's surface, another stunning feat.

Miller was an extremely meticulous researcher who had worked for almost ten years on the experiments he reported in 1969 (although several papers on parts of the data had appeared in the meantime). In this respect, he was very similar to Hans Berger. There was a major difference, though. Berger's EEG recordings and the modulation of brain waves by eye closure and mental activity were soon replicated in laboratories all over the world.

Conversely, Miller's biofeedback findings in paralysed animals could not even be replicated in his own laboratory, although he and his students tried for over 20 years, even setting up an "intensive care unit"[16] for rats. It is still not clear why these replication experiments failed. One possibility is that paralysing an animal and making it totally dependent on outside support abolishes all drive and motivation to engage in learning.

For most bio- or neurofeedback applications in humans, the question of whether preserved motor functions are a prerequisite for learning to control one's own physiology is a largely theoretical one. If biofeedback has positive effects on a person's clinical symptoms or well-being it does not matter to the patient exactly how it is achieved, and whether some element of motor training was involved. However, for completely locked-in patients who have lost all motor control because the higher centres in the brain are disconnected from the motor pathways (see Sections 1.1 and 1.2) the question of whether they can still be trained to modulate physiological signals to communicate with the outside world is of utmost importance. The big hope here relies on an approach that is available only with humans, where we can complement operant training with verbal instructions and thus utilise cognitive, potentially faster, learning mechanisms. For example, rather than trying to train a particular brain wave by trial and error, as one would in an animal experiment, we might be able to instruct a person to imagine moving their right or left hand and then read out the corresponding brain activation patterns. If successful, this could become a relatively easy and reliable tool for brain communication.

1.6   Brain computer interfaces and communication

The clinical studies of neurofeedback that started after Olds's and Fetz's seminal discoveries have shown that not only rats, cats and monkeys but also humans can learn to influence their brain rhythms. These clinical, therapeutic applications of neurofeedback will be the central theme of Chapter 3. For now we will focus on the use of brain training to enable communication. If a person can increase or decrease a brain wave, or shift its peak from one area to another, this could become a new way of expressing oneself, almost like learning a language. The necessary devices are called Brain Computer Interfaces (BCIs); they use brain signals, which can be picked up by EEG, for the control of an output device, for example a computer mouse. In order to enable a BCI to provide reliable output the patient needs to be able to influence his or her EEG signal with high accuracy. Because this is not a skill that we learn naturally, reliable control of the target signal has to be learned in the laboratory through some kind of neurofeedback procedure. Three features of the EEG signal have been mainly used for such communication BCIs, the slow cortical potentials, the sensorimotor rhythm and the P300 (as introduced in Section 1.4). Slow cortical potentials (SCP) are drifts in the EEG signal that have a low frequency (below 1 Hz) and can occur for several seconds during the preparation phase of mental or motor tasks. The sensorimotor rhythm (SMR) occurs in the lower beta range (12 Hz–20 Hz) and reflects oscillations between neurons in the thalamus and the somatosensory and motor cortices. It can be suppressed both by movements and by motor imagery, which also makes it an attractive target for self-regulation.

All BCIs include a series of steps for converting the measured brain signal into commands for a computer (Figure 1.8). Firstly, the relevant

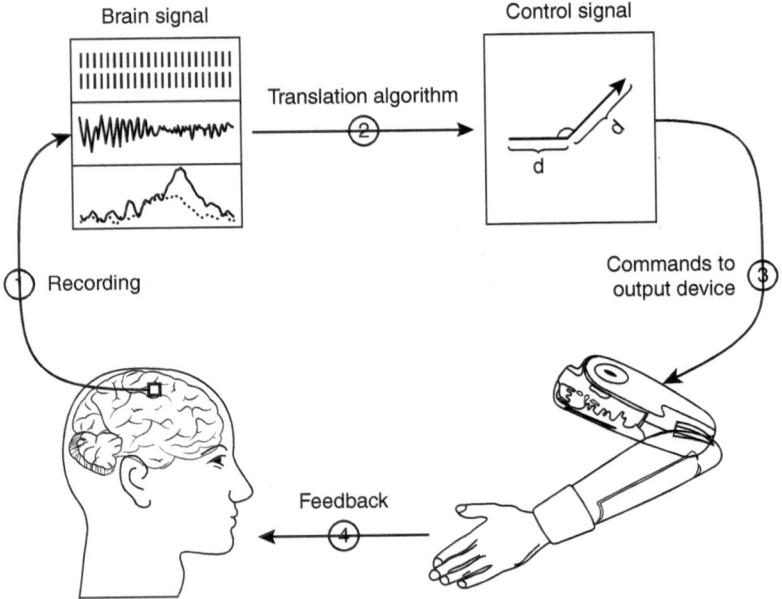

Figure 1.8   Basic diagram of a Brain Computer Interface, as described in text

Note: A recording device, for example EEG or electrodes inserted into the brain, picks up brain signals (1), which are analysed in real time. An algorithm extracts the relevant features, for example, the amplitude of the P300 wave. This parameter is converted into a control signal (2). This control signal is converted into commands to an external device, for example cursor movements on a computer screen or flexion and displacement of a robotic arm (3). In a complete feedback loop, the participant receives sensory feedback about this output and can learn to modulate it with his/her brain activity (4).

feature is extracted from the wealth of information that the measurement device picks up. If we take the example of the P300, this would entail filtering out some of the higher frequencies that can obscure the evoked potentials and computing the peak amplitude of the EEG around 300 ms after the stimulus presentation in relation to the preceding baseline. Of course, this analysis needs to happen as soon as possible after the event because robot control needs to be fast. Secondly, the extracted feature, in this case the P300 amplitude, needs to be converted into an output signal for the participant through a translation algorithm. In the simplest case, the computed amplitude can be converted linearly into the length of a bar or the position of a cursor on a computer screen, but if multiple features are extracted to enable a two- or three-dimensional output (e.g. for navigation of a wheelchair) more complex algorithms are needed. Finally, this translation from EEG feature to output needs to be adaptive. People's individual neurophysiological responses vary widely but still have to be projected onto the same computer screen. Thus, the conversion has to be adapted to an individual's response range. This principle applies to any training. If a novice athlete is to be rewarded for improved performance in the high jump there is no point in starting the cursor movement at 2 metres (6 ft 6'). This adaptation to the original signal also has to take into account the fluctuation of the signal over time, the improvement with training, and an individual's training capacity. For example, the duration of the training has to be adjusted to psychological factors like motivation and fatigue, which again corresponds to well known general principles from teaching and training.[17]

Amongst the EEG-based communication BCIs P300 spellers are most widely used and require the least amount of training of participants. P300 spellers work through the presentation of random sequences of letters or numbers on a computer screen. The participant wears a small set of EEG electrodes, which record the event-related potentials. He or she is asked to focus attention on the next intended character while ignoring all others. Modern computer algorithms can read out these intentions with high reliability from the presence or absence of P300 activity.[18] The speed of the speller can be improved further if the computer algorithm predicts the next likely letters and only presents the relevant ones. For example, if a person has already spelt "Good morni" it is likely that the next intended letter will be "n" and there is no need to present all 26 letters of the alphabet again.

For most people BCI communication is far too complicated because they have easier means of communication available. Even the most severely paralysed patients can communicate faster and more effectively through eye trackers or other motor devices than through a BCI. However, for patients in a completely locked-in state this avenue for communication would make a huge difference. This technique was pioneered by biological psychologist Niels Birbaumer's group, working at the University of Tübingen in Germany. They trained patients with MND to change the location of SCPs recorded on the scalp. Ultimately, some patients could actually spell letters by shifting their SCPs and write an entire letter (albeit over many weeks). Their initial report in the journal *Nature* in 1999[19] sparked much interest worldwide. Would locked-in patients finally be able to communicate, could their brains be un-locked? Other impressive achievements of almost totally paralysed patients include the computer artwork by Hhem, a 72-year old German artist who was diagnosed with MND in 2007. She uses a P300-BCI to select the shape, colour, position and size of objects on her paintings, producing images of wonderful complexity.[20] One of them featured on the cover of the neurology journal *Brain* in June 2013.

However, the researchers afterwards reported that they had not managed to train any patients who had lost the entire control of their motor functions.[16] However, these are the patients who would potentially benefit most from the BCI because those with preserved motor function can still communicate through eye or facial movements. Why has it so far been impossible to train completely locked-in patients with neurofeedback? Birbaumer and his colleague Leonardo Cohen, a neurologist working at the National Institutes of Health in the USA, have argued that the complete loss of control abolishes the motivational basis for any operant conditioning. According to this argument, those who cannot influence their muscles could not be expected to learn to control their brain. So how about training patients while they still have this sense of being able to influence their movements? This would not be possible for those who become suddenly locked-in after a stroke but would be possible for those with a gradual loss of motor functions in MND. Miller had shown that freely moving rats, trained to increase or decrease their heart rate to escape electric shocks, maintained this ability after being paralysed with curare. The analogy would be that patients with MND who learn to regulate their EEG while still in control of some of their muscles maintain this skill after they have lost all motor control. At present it is not known whether this would work, but it may be one avenue to brain communication in the locked-in state.

Another option to train brain responses for communication in completely locked-in patients may be the use of classical conditioning.

Birbaumer's group has recently tested this procedure in three patients with advanced MND, one of whom was in a completely locked-in state.[21] In training they paired correct statements, such as "Berlin is the capital of Germany", with electrical stimulation of the left thumb. The stimulation of the thumb, which reliably evokes specific potentials in the brain, was the unconditioned stimulus. The auditory presentation of the statement was the conditioned stimulus. The researchers presented an equal number of false statements, which were never paired with electrical stimulation. If we think back to the experiments on new motor connections performed by Doty and Giurgea, the goal of this approach is to train the brain to respond to true statements with the activation of the brain areas that normally only respond to stimulation of the thumb, without the need for pairing with electrical stimulation. In this way a yes answer could be read out from the presence of this thumb wave in response to a statement. Of course, the ultimate aim is not to find out whether completely locked-in patients know that Berlin is the capital of Germany but to enable them to communicate their feelings and wishes to their carers, or even to write letters or books as Jean-Dominique Bauby did with his blink code. However, the researchers' task was more complicated. The true statements did not evoke anything like a simple thumb wave in the EEG even after lengthy conditioning, and they had to use complex mathematical procedures to try and classify the brain responses into yes and no answers. Although such brain reading algorithms have been applied with reasonable accuracy in some experiments to decode people's intentions from their brain activity (see Section 1.8), this approach has not, so far, been successful in MND patients.

One of Birbaumer's patients, a 66-year old lady, developed a completely locked-in state only three years after the diagnosis of MND. Like all locked-in patients, she had to be artificially fed and ventilated. The researchers determined with EEG assessments that her brain distinguished between different types of information, for example rare and frequent stimuli of an oddball paradigm, and thus ascertained that she had preserved at least some cognitive functions. Overall, she received 37 daily sessions of the brain conditioning protocol. Even with this extensive training, though, her brain responses to true and false statements did not become sufficiently different to be read with currently available techniques. Thus, the problem of enabling completely locked-in patients to communicate through a BCI is still waiting for a solution.

An alternative to EEG for brain-based communication might be the use of methods that capture the vascular correlates of neural activity, such as functional magnetic resonance imaging (fMRI). The term imaging refers to techniques where physical processes are induced in the body and the effects, generally changes in electromagnetic radiation, can be picked up by a measurement device and allow for a reconstruction of two- or three-dimensional images of the respective body parts. Examples range from x-ray radiography to magnetic resonance imaging. Imaging becomes functional when the signal that is picked up by the technique is not just a static contrast between different tissue types (as in anatomical or structural imaging), but is dependent on chemical or electrical processes in the tissue. In the case of the brain, the functional processes that are picked up by functional neuroimaging are mainly the metabolism of glucose and oxygen, or differences in the binding of neurotransmitters and other signalling molecules. The first wave of functional neuroimaging techniques for use in humans, developed and refined in the 1960s–1980s, relied on radioactivity. By injecting patients or research participants with molecules that were radioactively labelled one could then trace the distribution of these molecules in the body by picking up the radioactivity emitted as the radioactive markers decayed. Several scanning techniques have been developed for this purpose, including single photon emission computed tomography (SPECT) and positron emission tomography (PET). They are still very important for the investigation of abnormalities in brain chemistry in patients with neurological and psychiatric disorders and to ascertain that drugs used for these disorders actually act in humans in the way predicted from animal studies.[22] However, their use to track changes in neural activity during specific mental processes (by looking at changes in glucose or oxygen consumption) has largely been superseded by the non-radioactive technique of fMRI, which was invented in the early 1990s. Functional MRI uses the same signal as anatomical MRI, which is based on the electromagnetic properties of the hydrogen atoms in body water and shows exquisite contrast between parts of the brain or other tissues at high spatial resolution. This MR signal is influenced by the oxygen saturation of the blood in neighbouring vessels. If the blood has given off its oxygen and its carrier molecule haemoglobin is thus de-oxygenised, it will attenuate the MR signal. The physical explanation is based on the paramagnetic properties of deoxy-haemoglobin, which introduce distortions in the local magnetic field, making it less homogeneous. Conversely, the oxy-haemoglobin that is carried with fresh blood, is diamagnetic (like water) and thus has no effects on the MR signal.

The net effect of an inflow of fresh, oxygenated blood into a part of the brain on the MR signal is thus positive, a signal increase. This component of the MR signal is called the blood oxygenation-level dependent (or BOLD) signal and, over the last 20 years, has become a very important surrogate marker of neural activity. Neural activity is an energy-demanding process that requires glucose and oxygen. The basic assumption behind the use of the BOLD signal for functional imaging is that increased neural activity, such as that evoked by a light flash in the visual areas of the brain, leads to changes in the local vessels that promote inflow of fresh blood. Because this supply of fresh blood exceeds what is needed to meet increased oxygen demands of the neural activity itself, it leads to a positive BOLD effect. Although this assumption does not hold in all cases (for example, it may not apply in patients with severe cerebral vessel disease) it is a reasonable starting point, and animal studies have confirmed the correspondence between the BOLD signal and some aspects of neuronal activity through direct cortical recordings during MR imaging.

The fMRI technique has been used widely over the past 20 years to map out the brain response to a wide variety of stimuli and the brain correlates of internal mental states, such as love, preferences for certain food or political allegiances (although not all of these could be replicated by other researchers). We used it in the late 1990s at the University of Frankfurt, Germany, to map out the neural activation underlying auditory hallucinations (voice hearing), a common and disturbing symptom of schizophrenia. We found that the same areas in the temporal lobe were active during hallucinations and when patients listened to another person speaking.[23]

Brain centres for hearing can thus be activated in the absence of any external stimulus. In fact, healthy individuals can obtain very similar results by merely imagining voices or sounds (auditory imagery).[24] Similarly, mere mental imagery of a movement can activate the same areas in the motor centres of the brain as the actual movement. It is well known that moving the right arm depends on activation of the left motor cortex (and vice versa for the left arm) and such lateralised activity also occurs when people just imagine moving their right or left arm.[25] This raises the exciting possibility of teaching patients to communicate by imagining particular movements. For example, they could imagine moving their right arm to signal yes and moving their left arm to signal no. In this way they could select letters from a display and thus "write" words or sentences. Although this brain computer interface would be similar to the EEG-based spelling devices it may be easier to operate because it is easier to instruct patients to imagine moving their right or left hand than to train them to regulate the notoriously capricious EEG signals. Such use of verbal instructions, which is obviously not available to animal experimentalists, can greatly speed up the learning procedure in humans. As explained, a simple device could just consist of left vs. right motor imagery to signal yes or no, but more sophisticated protocols with different types of imagery and mental activity are under development. The Latin alphabet used to spell English, and many other languages, has 26 letters, and if patients can learn to produce the corresponding number of brain states they could select letters from the full alphabet rather than just single letters at a time and thus greatly increase their "writing" speed. It may sound inconceivable to induce 26 nicely separable mental states that can be discriminated by the associated brain activity, but this feat has actually been achieved in healthy individuals. Bettina Sorger, a psychologist working at Maastricht University in the Netherlands achieved this by adding temporal information into the mix. By using three different durations (10, 20 and 30 seconds) and three different onset times she only needed three different mental tasks (inner speech, mental arithmetic and motor imagery) to achieve 27 (3×3×3) distinct states. Her participants could thus pick any letter from the alphabet (and one extra letter) in under one minute.[26] This is slow compared to normal writing, of course, but similar to the fastest EEG-based spelling devices. The researchers are now scanning MND patients in order to assess whether they, too, are capable of communicating in this way. The most interesting question, ultimately, will be whether fMRI-based communication can be achieved by completely locked-in patients.[27] The challenge will then be to take this technique into people's homes, which is obviously not possible with current MRI scanners. This is much easier for EEG, where home-based BCI devices are already on the market (mainly for neurofeedback and gaming). However, one of the technical cousins of fMRI, functional near-infrared spectroscopy (fNIRS), which also picks up blood oxygen signals but only from very superficial areas of the brain, could potentially be developed into such a bedside device.

1.7   Detecting conscious states

For patients with a clinical history of locked-in syndrome we assume that they can understand us and communicate with us if the appropriate technical aids can be provided. Their consciousness is not disturbed. However, there is another group of patients who do not communicate through normal means but who do in fact suffer from disorders of consciousness. Severe head trauma and other brain lesions, for example from anoxia (lack of oxygen supply), can initially lead to coma. This state resembles deep sleep, but even strong stimuli that would disrupt the sleep of anyone else (for example very loud sounds) cannot awaken these patients who may, at most, show reflex movements to pain. If a patient emerges from a coma but does not fully recover consciousness, two scenarios can emerge, persistent vegetative state (PVS) or minimally conscious state (MCS). Patients in PVS, also called unresponsive wakefulness syndrome, breathe independently, can have their eyes open and move spontaneously, but their movements are not targeted. They do not communicate and do not follow any commands but they do have an intact sleep-wake cycle. Patients with MCS respond variably and show some directed movements, but their communication is limited to simple gestures or verbal responses. Both PVS and MCS patients are bedbound and totally dependent on 24-hour care. Patients can stay in PVS or MCS for many years, but some can fully recover awareness even after years or decades. Determining the prognosis in these cases has been an important medical and ethical challenge for many years. One contested ethical issue is whether the essential life support, such as gastric tube feeding, may be withdrawn from patients who have practically no hope of regaining awareness. This debate took an unexpected turn several years ago when Adrian Owen, a Cambridge neuroscientist now based in London, Ontario in Canada, tested a patient with a presumed lack of awareness in the scanner. He asked the patient to imagine playing tennis. He reasoned that if the patient showed activation of the corresponding motor areas in the brain this would indicate that he understood the instructions. This is indeed what he observed. Thus the patient, who, according to his clinicians, was suffering from PVS or MCS, was fully aware and was more likely to be suffering from locked-in syndrome. These post-comatose patients are already suffering from a very disabling condition but it must make things even worse to be awake and aware while nobody takes any notice. A bigger study that Owen conducted with the Belgian neurologist Steven Laureys in patients with suspected PVS or MCS detected such imagery-related brain activity in about 10% of their patients, although they showed little or no outward signs of awareness.[28] This work was rightly hailed as providing an important new tool for the exploration and diagnosis of patients with disorders of consciousness (some of who may turn out to have no consciousness disorder at all, but just a severe disorder of communication, viz. the locked-in state). It may also open up the prospect of training patients to go beyond a simple imagery task and produce differential activation through which they can control a BCI and communicate, perhaps even use the Maastricht group's sophisticated spelling device that allows them to pick one letter out of the whole alphabet in a single attempt.

1.8   Reading thoughts directly from the brain

Another interesting approach would be to try and extract information about mental activity directly from brain activity without using an external BCI. In the examples given in Section 1.6 patients use their brain activity to move a cursor or to press a mouse button to pick a letter from a display, and thus essentially translate their thoughts and wishes into a set of mental activities that may not be directly related to their original thoughts but can be discriminated through brain imaging or EEG. For example, if they want to express the wish "I would like to watch football", they would have to go through a specific sequence of mental arithmetic and motor imagery to allow them to pick the relevant letters from the alphabet. It would be much quicker and easier for them – and would not require any training on the part of the patient – if the brain imaging device could read their thoughts and wishes directly from their brain activity. For example, if there is an area that lights up whenever I have a wish (but, and this is crucial, only then!), another area for "watch" and another for "football", a simple software programme could extract the meaning from the brain activation. In reality, this is bound to be much harder because there are few, if any, such highly specific brain areas. The brain activation associated with the wish to watch football is much more muddled than this ideal scenario of three nicely separate areas becoming active at the same time. However, in principle – and if the resolution of the imaging technique is fine-grained enough – it should be possible to identify the activation patterns associated with specific thoughts. This field of research, which has grown enormously over the last decade and is sometimes also termed brain reading, uses sophisticated statistical techniques and computer algorithms to discriminate the brain states associated with specific mental states.[29] The crucial test is then whether the identified brain state predicts the mental state accurately (in the same person, or even in another). Let us assume that one of these algorithms is trained to discriminate between my brain activation patterns associated with "I want to watch football" and "I want to have tea", based on my thoughts during an imaging experiment. When I am next in the scanner, the researchers will wait for similar brain activation patterns to emerge and tell me that I must be hungry or wanting to watch football. If they predicted my mental states accurately I would be convinced that their algorithm worked (and that the brain imaging was fine-grained enough). For the participant this task is easy – just think your thoughts – but for the algorithm it involves a considerable amount of training and, thus far, computer programmes have only been able to predict people's mental states with an accuracy around 60%–70%, and only in fairly controlled laboratory settings. One problem for clinical applications is that the algorithms always have to be trained on the to-be-discriminated mental states first and it is unknown how well they can then generalise and predict new mental states. But for patients whose range of interaction with the environment is limited anyway, such as those with complete paralysis, it may be very useful to have trained an algorithm to understand a small set of commands, such as "Open the window", "Lift my bed" or "Switch off the light". One general limitation with this automatic brain reading approach is that even if it works in the laboratory it will be very difficult to translate it to the bedside because extracting the complex activation patterns of specific thoughts is likely to require high resolution measurements, such as those obtained by fMRI or even invasive recordings. Bedside devices such as simple electrode caps or NIRS sensors are more suited to picking up simple yes/no responses.

1.9   The brain controls a robot

Let us explore these thoughts further. If a computer algorithm can read my wish to have the light switched off from my brain activity, its use would not be confined to telling an experimenter or carer about my wishes, it could also switch off the light directly. What is required for these types of application is an interface between my brain readout and a robot. Many engineers are working on such brain-driven robots, and the Japanese car manufacturer Honda has developed a robot that can be instructed to execute a number of preselected actions by participants who have trained the respective EEG patterns through neurofeedback. Along similar lines, Honda's competitors Toyota have developed a wheelchair whose controls are operated through EEG signals. Self-regulation of EEG signals, though, does not allow for many degrees of freedom and it is unlikely that people can learn to evoke more than two or three specific states. Up until now it has not been possible to achieve the detailed readouts of brain activity needed to control robots or prosthetic devices in everyday situations using those EEG, fMRI or other techniques that do not require surgical placement of electrodes (so-called non-invasive techniques). However, researchers can read out motor plans from dense electrode arrays that are inserted invasively into the motor cortex (Figure 1.8).[30] Most of this work has been conducted in monkeys. It has been known for a while that specific groups, or populations, of nerve cells in the motor areas of the brain control movement in specific directions. If we can record from these nerve cells during sessions where a monkey freely moves its arm in different directions, we can then train an algorithm to identify the neural signatures of specific movements, and not just simple movements, such as reaching to a position on a touch-screen, but also more complex ones, such as grasping an object and putting it into the mouth. These signals can then be used to control a robot that performs just these actions. This is not just an interesting technical challenge but would also have enormous health benefits if the same could be achieved in patients who still produce these motor signals in their brains but lack the limbs to execute them, or whose communication pathways from brain to limb are disturbed, as in spinal injuries or in the locked-in state as the most extreme example.

One spectacular report on two monkeys who managed to control a robot with their thoughts was published by a group of researchers from Pittsburgh in 2008 in the journal *Nature*.[31] The researchers connected an artificial arm to a computer that read signals from the monkeys' motor areas. The monkeys managed to use this arm prosthesis to execute a rather complex movement, picking up a marshmallow from the experimenter's hand and putting it into the mouth. Apparently, they also considered the arm prosthesis to be part of their body because they started licking it as if it was their own arm. Such a sense of the robot as an extension of one's own body is likely to be very important for seamless use in everyday settings. The fluidity of robotic movements is still very far from being satisfactory. Although the monkeys managed to grasp the pieces of food and put them into their mouths, they took much longer than with real movements, often had to adjust their movement half-way and were not successful on all attempts.

One reason for the limited success of brain-controlled prostheses may be that although the motor control achieved by a BCI may be rather good, it crucially lacks the direct sensory feedback that continually guides our actions. If we bang our hand against a hard surface we immediately feel pain, whereas in a BCI experiment one just gets the rather abstract feedback that one has failed the trial or, in the case of the monkeys described above, notice that the marshmallow has slipped out of the hand. One solution might be to feed back the sensory consequences of the corresponding actual (rather than robotic) movement. One way of doing this would be to connect the BCI to a device (orthosis) that moves the appropriate arm passively. Such devices are actually in use for neurofeedback trials in stroke rehabilitation, but in humans have only supported very simple movements.[32] Another option would be to keep delivering the output through the artificial limb but simulate the sensory consequences of the real movement. Because the main clinical target group, spinal cord injury patients, have generally lost the transmission of both motor and sensory signals, attaching stimulators to the real limb would not be sufficient, so the sensory consequences of the movement, such as hitting an object, need to be fed back directly to the brain. The group of Miguel Nicolelis, working at Duke University in the USA and at the University of Natal in Brazil, is spearheading the development of such brain–machine–brain interfaces in monkeys.[33]

Another option to make brain-controlled movements feel more natural would be to connect the BCI directly to the paralysed muscles, which has already been achieved in monkeys. As published in *Nature* 2008, the group of Eberhard Fetz, the pioneer of monkey neurofeedback, trained monkeys to flex their wrist through neurofeedback, using electrical signals from single nerve cells in motor cortex. They silenced the normal neural input into the wrist muscles by injecting a local anaesthetic, but implanted into the paralysed muscles electrodes that were under the control of the BCI.[34] Thus, monkeys controlled the hand movements through the practised brain activity, which was directly linked to the output muscle, bypassing the natural motor pathways that travel through the brainstem, spinal cord and peripheral nerves. Although in these monkeys the successful muscle control was merely a technological achievement, it could have real practical implications for patients with spinal or peripheral nerve injuries. These patients have preserved functions of the motor cortex and the muscles and limbs but lack the communication between them. They would therefore benefit particularly from such a "neuroprosthesis".[35]

The first successful trial of a brain-robot control interface in humans made the news internationally in May 2012. The group of researchers around John Donoghue and Leigh Hochberg at Brown University in Providence, Rhode Island, USA had been working for many years with a small number of patients with stroke or spinal cord injury. All these patients were tetraplegic, meaning that they could not control any of their limbs, and they had electrodes surgically implanted into the upper limb area of their motor cortex. The surgeons implanted arrays of 96 silicon electrodes that reached 1.5 mm into the cortical area. The first challenge was to ensure that the electrodes stayed functional over many years by making them as biocompatible as possible.[36] The next challenge was to train the computer algorithm to recognise movement intentions from the brain signals. The researchers achieved this step in 2006 when they demonstrated that humans could control a computer cursor with their thoughts.[37] It took them another six years to develop a robotic interface and train patients to use it, but in 2012 they had finally demonstrated that two patients could move an artificial arm through their motor cortex activity. One patient even managed to move a cup to her mouth and drink from it, which she had been unable to do for 15 years after being paralysed by a midbrain stroke. Although it was to be expected that humans could learn these skills if monkeys could, it was not at all clear that patients who had been tetraplegic for many years would still be able to modulate their motor cortex activity with the appropriate imageries. This report[38] was therefore welcomed as a major medical breakthrough, and was carried on newspapers, news sites, radio and television programmes all over the globe. It gave the hope of regaining some level of independence to the hundreds of thousands of patients worldwide paralysed after spinal cord injury. For example, it may ultimately be possible for them to control a wheelchair and feed themselves with the power of their thoughts. Although this would require them to have their brains wired up permanently to a BCI, this would probably be a price many of them would be prepared to pay.

2
External Control of the Brain: Brain Stimulation and Psychiatric Surgery

2.1 Fits and faints: the network out of control

> We have often seen someone constrained on a sudden by the violence of disease, who, as if struck by a thunderbolt, falls to the ground, foams at the mouth, groans and shudders, raves, grows rigid, twists, pants irregularly, outwearies himself with contortions.[39]

This classic description of an epileptic fit is more than 2,000 years old but could still feature in a modern textbook of clinical neurology. It was provided by the Roman poet Lucretius in the 1st century BC in a poem in which he sought to describe phenomena of the animate and inanimate world in materialistic terms. The point that epilepsy was a disease of the body, more specifically of the brain, had already been made 400 years before by the Greek doctor Hippocrates in his slim book on *The Sacred Disease* (which he did not consider to be sacred or god-given at all). Lucretius's point was that if the mind is so readily clouded by a disease of the body (and cure of that disease restores its clarity) it could not have the independent existence that many philosophers claimed for it. According to Lucretius, the mind can only be changed by changing its material substrate. This idea is still very much alive in debates on the mind-body problem today, and is even relevant to psychiatry and neuroscience. For example, psychiatrists and psychologists have been trying to change patients' minds through psychological interventions, such as psychoanalysis or cognitive behavioural therapy, for over 100 years, but the idea that psychotherapy might work through changes in the brain was still a controversial proposition only a few years ago.[40]

In addition to its philosophical importance, Lucretius's description of epilepsy is also very useful to historians of medicine because it suggests that the clinical presentation of epilepsy has not changed much over the centuries. He describes the sudden onset, initial loss of body tone, shaking of the limbs or the whole body, and rigidity that are typical of what today's clinicians would call tonic-clonic or, using a 19th century French term, Grand mal seizures. Tonic describes the shift between loss of muscle tone and heightened tone (rigidity), and clonic describes the involuntary, high frequency movements. During these seizures, patients often lose consciousness, they might bite their tongue or pass urine or stool, a phenomenon already recognised by Hippocrates, who was also an astute clinical observer. These Grand mal seizures usually only last for up to a few minutes, but they can usher in a prolonged state of convulsions and loss of consciousness. Grand mal seizures, and particularly the longer Grand mal states, are feared because patients can get into breathing difficulties and suffer brain damage from lack of oxygen. In addition, they often hurt themselves when falling or hitting sharp objects. Uncontrolled epilepsy also severely constrains patients in their daily lives. They are generally not allowed to drive cars or operate machinery, which excludes them from many jobs. They also need to take precautions to minimise their risk of injury, such as wearing helmets or padding their homes. Another problem is that, in time, their memory and other cognitive abilities can decline, probably because of damage to the brain from uncontrolled electrical activity underlying the seizures and from restrictions to local oxygen supply. Many patients also develop psychiatric problems.

Until the early 20th century medicine did not have much to offer patients suffering from epilepsy, but the introduction of barbiturates and more advanced anti-epileptic or anticonvulsant drugs brought about very good control of seizures – both acutely and in the long term – for the majority of epilepsy patients. Epileptic seizures arise when the delicate balance between inhibitory and excitatory circuits in a brain network is disturbed and activity can spread unchecked, and anti-epileptic drugs aim to stabilise the nerve cell membrane and shift the balance back to inhibitory activity. However, up to 40% of patients with epilepsy do not respond to the available drugs, and even combinations of drugs fail to control their seizures. This is still a considerable number because epilepsy is common, for example, it affects about 2 million people in the USA. Some of these treatment-refractory patients are potential candidates for epilepsy surgery. The idea behind surgical intervention for epilepsy is that, if there is a focus in the brain from which the seizure activity originates, removing it might control the fits. The idea of a focus is supported by the observation that many Grand mal seizures start with convulsions of a specific body part. In fact, some seizures may remain focal and confined to the involuntary movement of one limb, for example the right arm, without any impairment of consciousness. In this case one would suspect a focus in the left motor cortex. Similarly, if a patient only experiences sensations in the right arm one would suspect a focus in the left somatosensory cortex. Seizures which are confined to one functional system are called focal, or partial, whereas those that seem to affect large parts of the brain, as evidenced by convulsions of limbs on both sides accompanied by particular electrical patterns in the EEG, are called generalised. Some partial seizures are characterised by more complex patterns of behaviour than just movement or sensation in one limb. During these complex partial seizures patients may walk around aimlessly or engage in repetitive, stereotyped movements. Although they are awake and may stare at others they are unresponsive and later have no recollection of the event. The location of the focus of such complex partial seizures was initially not as obvious as that of simple motor or sensory seizures, but we now know that it resides in the temporal lobe in most cases. Until the discovery of the EEG, which can pick up the electrical activity associated with seizures through the skull, physicians had to diagnose epilepsy based on the clinical presentation of the patient alone. However, if an operation to remove the focus from the brain is contemplated, the suspected location of the focus has to be verified with invasive recordings, where neurosurgeons place electrodes inside the brain to record over several weeks, because the resolution of the conventional scalp EEG is not sufficient. This approach was pioneered by the neurophysiologist Reginald Bickford in the 1940s and 1950s, first at Oxford and later at the Mayo Clinic in Rochester, New York. When they open the skull to insert recording electrodes neurosurgeons also have the opportunity to stimulate specific areas of the brain in order to establish their function (and avoid damaging them in the course of the surgery). The Canadian neurosurgeon Wilder Penfield conducted groundbreaking studies on the brain correlates of consciousness and personal memories with this approach in the 1940s and 1950s, which will be presented in detail in Section 2.3.

2.2 Limbic circuits: memory and emotions in the brain

Even without direct recordings from the brain one might suspect that complex partial seizures are generated in the temporal lobes of the brain.

They are often preceded by, so-called, auras, during which patients hear voices of people they used to know, relive experiences from their past, or just have the illusion of having experienced something before (déjà vu). Both hearing and memory are functions of the temporal lobe. Furthermore, during the period of impaired consciousness patients may engage in inappropriate behaviours, which can even take an aggressive turn. After the event, they have no memory of these actions. Aggression and fear are mediated through areas in the limbic system, which comprises parts of the temporal lobes as well. The Latin word *limbus* means border, and the brain areas in question (Figure 2.1) border the lateral ventricles, the big fluid-filled cavities in the two hemispheres.

The limbic system was recognised as harbouring some of the brain's older (in evolutionary terms) functions, those of emotion and memory, by American doctors James Papez and Paul MacLean in the 1930s to 1950s. A particularly striking demonstration of the relevance for memory of one of its parts, the hippocampus, was obtained when epilepsy sufferer Henry Molaison had his hippocampus (and adjacent areas in the medial temporal lobe) removed on both sides by neurosurgeon William Scoville in 1953. This procedure cured his epilepsy but left

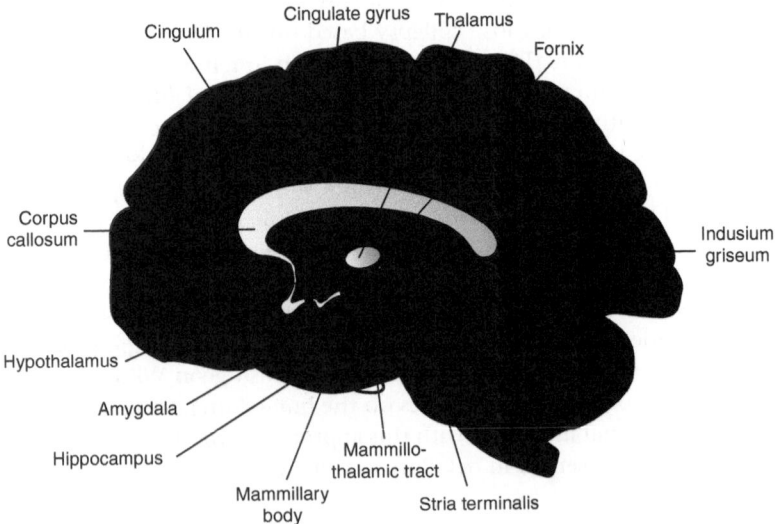

Figure 2.1   Location of the limbic system, its main components and adjacent areas

Note: Many of these areas have been targets for psychiatric surgery and Deep Brain Stimulation (DBS).

him unable to form new memories (most of his memories for the time before the operation and his ability to speak English were preserved). Many subsequent studies have highlighted the importance of the hippocampus and its connections for the storage of memories about life events, the so-called episodic memory. In 1937, Papez had described a memory circuit that travelled from the hippocampus around the limbic system and included the thalamus and the mammillary bodies. This last structure is of great interest to memory researchers because its destruction leads to Korsakoff's syndrome. This syndrome is classically associated with alcohol abuse, although the destruction of the mammillary bodies is not caused directly by the alcohol consumption but by the inadequate diet of many chronic alcohol abusers and lack of vitamin B1 intake. Korsakoff's syndrome differs somewhat from the memory loss (or amnesia) observed after hippocampal damage. Its classic feature is confabulation, where gaping holes in the patient's own memory are filled with plausible but fabricated information.

The role of the limbic system in emotions and emotional behaviour was postulated based on a large body of animal experiments demonstrating that the amygdala is relevant for emotional learning. Of course, we do not really know what an animal feels but can infer its emotional state from the way it behaves. A classical way to study this is through fear conditioning protocols in rodents. For example, if a tone that is primarily not aversive is regularly paired with an electric shock, this tone alone will, after a while, evoke a startle response in a rat. We might infer that the rat is afraid of the upcoming electric shock; it has established a fear memory. Damage to the amygdala reduces the strength of such fear conditioning. This can obviously make the animal less capable of detecting danger. In monkeys, who are eminently social animals, amygdala lesions can reduce the ability to behave appropriately towards other group members. Destruction of the amygdala can furthermore produce problems with memory and visual recognition of objects. It can also lead to severe behavioural changes, with increased sexual libido, overeating and the compulsory tendency to put things in the mouth (called hyperorality). This symptom complex was first observed by psychologist Heinrich Klüver and neurosurgeon Paul Bucy when they lesioned the temporal lobes of monkeys in the 1930s; it was also reported later in human patients. Although the evidence from human studies on the relevance of the amygdala for emotions and social interaction is not clear cut, there have been studies on the small number of patients with isolated damage to the amygdala. For example, in a genetic condition called Urbach-Wiethe syndrome parts of the medial temporal lobe are calcified and lose function. Some of the affected patients have an impaired ability to recognise fear in others and are also generally fearless themselves.

The limbic system is also tightly coupled with the brain's reward and motivation system. The neurotransmitter most strongly implicated in reward-based learning is dopamine. Dopamine is produced by a group of nerve cells, called dopaminergic neurons, that make up only a very small proportion of the brain's cells. However, they are crucial for several key functions, including learning and motor control, and loss of these neurons can lead to Parkinson's disease and other movement disorders. Once dopamine has been released by a nerve cell it binds to receptors on other neurons, where it can trigger a variety of chemical effects (Figure 2.2). It can also bind to the neuron from where it was released and thus block the release of further dopamine, establishing a negative feedback loop. Another way of controlling the amount of dopamine in the space between neurons, the synaptic cleft, is through the activity of the dopamine transporter, which moves dopamine back into the releasing neuron. The dopamine transporter is an important target for drugs for attention deficit/hyperactivity disorder (ADHD), such as methylphenidate and also for drugs of abuse, such as amphetamine. These drugs block the dopamine transporter and thus extend the lifetime of dopamine in the synaptic cleft, enhancing its biological effects.

Nerve cells in the ventral tegmental area (VTA) in the midbrain are important dopaminergic neurons. These VTA neurons are connected with several limbic areas, including the amygdala and the hippocampus, and with a part of the basal ganglia called the ventral striatum. This group of projections is called the mesolimbic pathway because it connects the midbrain (mesencephalon) with the limbic system. It is crucial for reward-based learning. One of the possible reasons for the difficulty training completely locked-in patients in instrumental control over their brain activity (Section 1.6) may be that neural damage in these patients had reached the dopaminergic cells of the midbrain.

2.3   History of brain stimulation

Cortical stimulation in humans

Much of our knowledge about the function of the cerebral hemispheres and the limbic system derives from direct electrical stimulation studies. The link between electrical stimulation and muscle activity was known since the 18th century when the Italian physician Luigi Galvani observed that direct electrical stimulation caused contractions in "frogs" legs. Links between specific brain areas and specific muscle

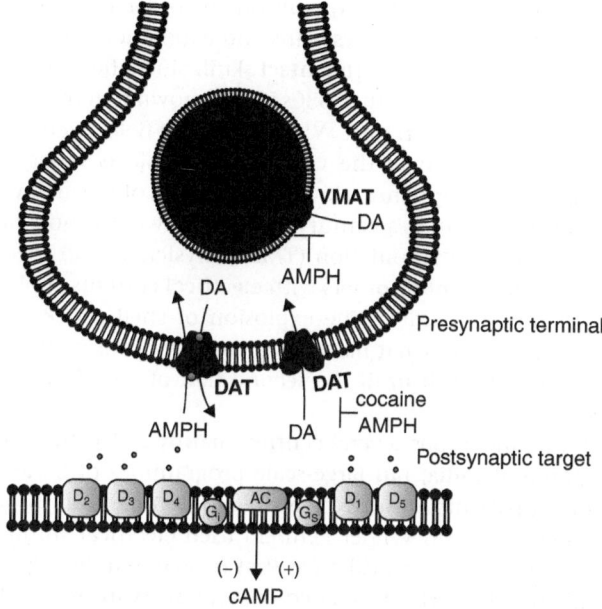

Figure 2.2 The dopaminergic synapse

Note: The upper part of the figure shows a synaptic terminal of a dopaminergic neuron with a storage vesicle. Several mechanisms by which drugs enhance dopamine activity are shown: Amphetamine (AMPH) reverses the dopamine (DA) transport into the presynaptic cell by acting as a substrate for the dopamine transporter (DAT) and blocks its storage by blocking the vesicular monoamine transporter (VMAT). Cocaine is also an inhibitor of dopamine reuptake into the cell. As a consequence, more dopamine remains in the cleft between the two neurons and can act onto the second, "postsynaptic" neuron. The lower part shows the postsynaptic membrane with the five types of dopamine receptor. Dopamine receptors can be coupled to inhibitory (D2–D4) or stimulating (D1, D5) G-proteins, resulting in decrease or increase of cyclic adenosine monophosphate (cAMP). Cyclic AMP is a "second messenger" molecule, which influences a wide variety of cellular processe. The different properties of dopamine receptors explain why dopamine can have so many different effects on behaviour. Adapted from figures 6.6. and 7.5 of Linden, *The Biology of Psychological Disorders*.[5]

groups were established in the 1870s by German neurologist Eduard Hitzig and physiologist Gustav Fritsch. They induced movements by direct electrical stimulation of the brain of dogs who were awake and their findings were later confirmed in monkeys by the leading English physiologist Charles Sherrington. Although evolution was still a new concept (Darwin's *On the Origin of Species* was first published in 1859), most physicians and scientists assumed that similar processes must be at play in humans, and indeed this was confirmed in 1893 when German neurosurgeon Fedor Krause mapped out the motor strip of a 15-year old girl who suffered from motor convulsions in order to find the lesion responsible for her epilepsy. Physicians and experimentalists soon tried to stimulate the brain through the intact skull. Since the work of English physicist Michael Faraday in the 1830s it was known that magnetic fields could induce electrical currents. When magnetic fields were applied to the back of the brain, over the visual areas, subjects reported seeing flashes of light, or phosphenes. However, this field of research was abandoned, and it took almost a century to develop what is now known as Transcranial Magnetic Stimulation (TMS). Physicians also tried to cure patients with movement disorders with electrical currents applied to the skull, for example to address the explosion of shell shock during the First World War. Again, what has become today's Transcranial Electrical Stimulation, had to wait until the second half of the 20th century for further development.

In the 1950s and 1960s several centres, mainly in North America but also in Japan and India, ran large-scale programmes of invasive brain stimulation in patients with psychiatric and neurological disorders. In Montreal, neurosurgeon Wilder Penfield used electrical stimulation to explore the function of cortical areas that he exposed during surgery to remove epileptic foci. He stimulated cortical areas in over a thousand patients. About half of them had suspected foci in the temporal lobes. Dramatic effects could be obtained by electrical stimulation of language areas:

> If the patient tried to speak while the electrode was in place, he discovered to his astonishment (and to ours at first) that he could not find his words. If shown a pencil, he knew what it was and could make appropriate movements with the hand, but he had lost the power of speaking. ... But as the electrode was lifted, the patient, not knowing what had been done, would exclaim, "Now I can speak. That was a pencil!".[41]

Depending on the stimulated region, Penfield could also induce patients to relive episodes from their past and even develop full-blown hallucinations, for example, hearing familiar voices or songs that were popular during their childhood. One patient who had grown up in a Dutch, art-loving family reported hallucinating about Rembrandt's famous painting *The Nightwatch*. However, the patients were always aware that these experiences were not real. These types of very vivid experiences, which are however recognised as not corresponding to stimuli from the outside world, would be called pseudohallucinations today, to distinguish them from the hallucinations of psychotic patients (and some epileptic patients during seizures). Penfield's patients also reported experiences of déjà-vu during stimulation, which are characterised by the firm conviction of having experienced a particular situation before when it is actually not the case. Such experiences are also reported by epilepsy patients during seizures.

When Penfield analysed his series of over a thousand patients he realised that he could alter mental states with electrical stimulation of areas in the temporal cortex in about 7% of patients, but not with stimulation of other brain areas.

Musical hallucinations were most commonly reported by Penfield's patients, followed by other auditory and visual experiences, and gustatory (taste) and olfactory (smell) hallucinations. Some patients became dazed. The experiences reported by the patients under brain stimulation were generally similar to those they reported during seizures or in the run-up to seizures, during the so-called auras. This suggests that Penfield was often stimulating areas that actually contributed to the seizures and were therefore altered by epilepsy. Thus, we cannot necessarily infer from these studies that patients not suffering from epilepsy would react in exactly the same way. It is interesting that Penfield's stimulation mainly induced re-experience of (often forgotten) events from the patient's past, rather than producing completely novel experiences. For example, a 25-year old French Canadian, who had suffered seizures with hallucinations since he was 19, "heard" a familiar song, "Oh Marie, Oh Marie" (a Neapolitan song which became the theme tune of the popular American radio comedy *Life with Luigi*) during stimulation of the right temporal plane.

> He explained that he had heard this before. "It is a theme song", he said, "on a radio program. The program is called the *Life of Luigi*," The patient...ended by singing the well-known refrain "Oh Marie, Oh Marie." All in the operating room recognised the song.[42]

A 22-year old man who had left South Africa a month before described the effects of stimulation of his superior temporal gyrus as follows:

> Now I hear people laughing – my friends in South Africa.[42]

Another example of temporal lobe stimulation that evoked very vivid sensory memories was the case of a 17-year old boy from the epilepsy programme of the American National Institute of Neurological Diseases and Blindness.[43] This boy had suffered brain damage from lack of oxygen at birth. For about two years he had been suffering from frequent seizures. When an electrode was inserted about two centimetres into his left temporal lobe he said that he "felt 6 years old again". When the electrode was moved a bit he reported having "a sensation like I was building a jet-racer", which was red and blue. Later, he reported seeing himself deer hunting with his father. Both experiences actually related to real events from his past. Three years before the operation he had built a soap-box car, and four years before he had been deer hunting with his father.

From what we know about the network structure of the brain, one could have predicted that electrical stimulation would trigger a re-experiencing of memory rather than creating a completely new experience. Memories are not stored in a single location in the brain and conscious experiences are not produced by activation of a single area. Many specialised modules have to work in a coordinated fashion and form networks to produce a specific sensory experience. Destruction of a single brain area – a single node of such a network – can destroy a memory or sensory experience. This sometimes happens in patients suffering from traumatic brain injury who develop retrograde amnesia, the loss of memory for events before the accident. However, the converse is not true, stimulation of a single node cannot bring about the experience of a complex mental state, unless it co-activates the rest of the network. These focal stimulations in all likelihood triggered activation of pre-formed networks and thus recreated the specific experiences or hallucinations reported by the patients.

However, as the American psychologist and historian of neuroscience Elliot Valenstein had pointed out 40 years ago,[44] this by no means implies that the experiences induced by the stimulation of a particular brain region are completely determined and always the same. One reason is the technical difficulty of replicating exactly a previous brain stimulation protocol. Another, even more fundamental, reason is that brain networks are dynamic and altered by every single experience, even by that of a preceding brain stimulation experiment. Furthermore, the effects of any stimulation will be influenced by the environment and setting in which they happen and by the patient's mood and concerns on each individual day. What remains, thus, is the prevailing observation that cortical stimulation, for all its dramatic power to induce altered states of consciousness, rarely produces experiences that are completely new to the patient but does trigger hallucinations of previous events.

This was certainly the model that Penfield himself applied in order to understand the meaning of the experiences that he triggered electrically. Penfield recounts the case of a 12-year old boy who received temporal lobe stimulation and reported the following experience:

> "Oh, gee, gosh, robbers are coming at me with guns!" He heard nothing, he just saw them coming at him. The robbers seemed to have been coming at an angle from the left. When asked if they came in front of him, he said no they were behind him.[42]

Penfield did not attribute this memory hallucination to an actual past experience of being threatened by robbers but to reading about this in the past.

> This seems to be the reproduction not of a real event, but of a fantasy or a dream drawn from the reading of a comic book. [42]

Penfield did not entertain the alternative explanation that the patient was having a completely new emotional experience, for example, by forming associations between what he knew about robbers and visual images of familiar people. Penfield felt cortical stimulation was re-evoking past mental states rather than creating new ones.

The effects of electrical stimulation of subcortical areas were even more dramatic than the hallucinatory experiences induced by temporal lobe stimulation. Subcortical areas include the brain regions covered by the large cortical mantles of the two hemispheres of the brain, which are therefore harder to access. In some cases Penfield had stimulated the amygdala and surrounding areas of the limbic system (see Section 2.2) and evoked automatisms, periods of automatic behaviour and confusion, for which the patient subsequently had no memory. Again, these episodes were indistinguishable from seizures generated by these areas, the psychomotor or complex partial seizures of temporal lobe epilepsy. Penfield's occasional observation that he could induce complex motor acts, similar to those observed in temporal lobe epilepsy, by limbic stimulation suggested that brain stimulation could induce not only experiences but also behaviours. The neurosurgeons of the late 19th century had induced limb movements through stimulation of the motor cortex. Similarly, simple movement, such as thumb twitching, can be induced by applying strong magnetic fields over the motor area of the human brain. These movements are then not under our control and if we try and suppress them we might only make them even stronger. Such loss of motor control may be perceived by some as a threat to their personal identity. This becomes an even more prominent issue if the electromagnetic stimulation directly influences brain centres that govern more complex, and perhaps personal, behavioural programmes. Whether such behavioural, or mind, control is possible – and desirable – with brain stimulation will be one of the central recurring themes of this book. Before we can turn to the evidence on this question from human studies we need to trace the history of the more detailed brain stimulation studies in animals.

Subcortical stimulation/self stimulation in animals

The subcortical areas are generally more similar in animals and humans than the cerebral cortex, which is much more developed in humans even more than in our closest relatives, the great apes. We need to appreciate the difficulty of comparing the brains of different species, which can vary in size by a factor of 1,000 (between mouse and human) and even more if we consider the much smaller brains of insects, which can provide important insights into neural function as well. For research that is intended to model stimulation effects on the human brain other vertebrates are the main target. Regardless of the differences in size and specialisation, the vertebrate brain has some general features that are constant across all species. It has six parts: the medulla, pons, cerebellum, midbrain, diencephalon and cerebrum (Figure 1.6). The medulla, pons and midbrain are often collectively termed the brainstem. We have already encountered the cerebrum and its sheet of nerve cells, the cerebral cortex, as the seat of many higher functions, including our memories for past events, through the stimulation work of Penfield. The cortex sends commands and receives input from the periphery through the long fibre tracts travelling through the midbrain, pons and medulla. As we saw in Chapter 1, if these communication tracts are destroyed paralysis and severe communication difficulties can result. These areas also contain important relay and control centres, for example: the substantia nigra in the midbrain, important for movement adjustment; the nuclei of cranial nerves in the pons, which relay the motor and sensory functions of the head and neck; and centres for breathing in the medulla. The diencephalon contains another important relay station, the thalamus, which has been termed the gatekeeper to the cerebral cortex. Most fibres that convey sensory input from the periphery (visual, auditory, tactile) have their terminus in the thalamus, which then distributes the incoming information to the appropriate specialised fields in the cerebral cortex.

Another main structure of the diencephalon is the hypothalamus, which controls many basic processes of life such as body temperature, sleep/wake cycles and food intake (Figure 2.3). It releases hormones, for example, oxytocin, which is primarily relevant for the regulation of pregnancy and milk production but has also been suspected to be a factor in the general disposition of the human species to be social. In addition to direct hormone release, the hypothalamus also controls the release of hormones from the pituitary gland. These hormones regulate the core bodily functions of growth, metabolism (conversion of food into energy) and procreation.

The hypothalamus is also a central control station for the vegetative, or autonomic, nervous system. So far we have encountered two of the three main parts of the nervous system, the central (brain and spinal cord) and the peripheral (nerves connecting the brainstem and spinal cord with muscles and sensory receptors in the periphery). The autonomic nervous system carries this name because it is generally not under voluntary control and has to keep operating in an undisturbed manner during both sleep and effortful mental activity. It connects the central nervous system with internal organs, such as the heart, blood vessels and guts. It has two parts, the sympathetic and the parasympathetic nervous systems, which have partly opposing functions. The parasympathetic

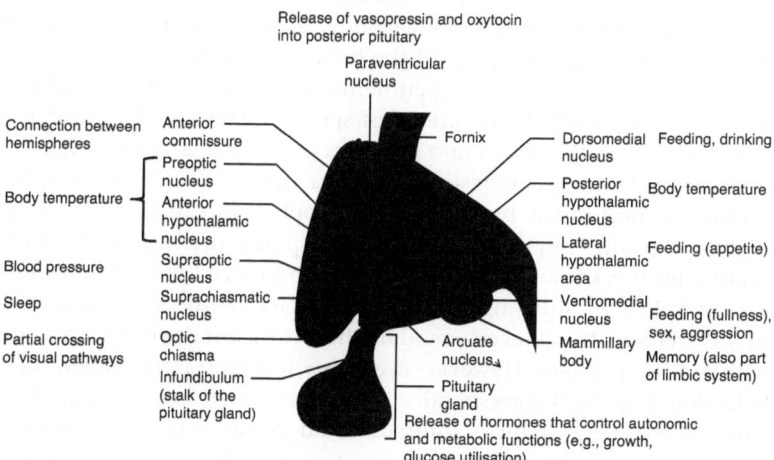

Figure 2.3 Nuclei of the hypothalamus and their main functions

Note: Note that some of the presumed functions (particularly control of aggression and sexual behaviour) are mainly inferred from comparative work in other animals, such as cats.

system supports the activities related to the internal housekeeping of the body, such as digesting food or voiding the bladder. Conversely, when an animal has to fight, flee or hunt prey, the sympathetic system becomes active and shifts activity from the digestive system to the heart and lungs.

The first researcher who systematically investigated the physiological and behavioural effects of the stimulation of deep brain areas in awake animals was the Swiss neurophysiologist Walter Rudolph Hess (1881–1973). Starting in the 1920s he conducted a large-scale research programme on the effects of the stimulation of the hypothalamus of cats. Focal stimulation of hypothalamic areas affected basic physiological responses, such as heart rate, blood pressure or temperature regulation, and could induce sleep. However, Hess also reported dramatic changes in an animal's behaviour after stimulation of specific parts of the hypothalamus. For example, in his Nobel Lecture of 1949 he described how "a formerly good-natured cat turns bad-tempered". He had managed, through electrical stimulation alone, to induce the behavioural pattern corresponding to a cat's response to a dog, including spitting, trying to attack and general physiological arousal.

The German biologist Erich von Holst, working in the 1950s, used electrical stimulation of specific brain regions to alter the behaviour of chickens. For example, by stimulating a certain area in the brainstem he triggered all the behaviours that occur when the chicken flees from an approaching predator – gaggling, running about, finally flying up. By stimulating other parts of the brainstem he triggered feeding or mating behaviours.[45] These experiments provided impressive evidence of the degree to which alterations of specific brain circuits can determine behaviour. Von Holst and his colleagues also managed to modify natural behaviours in interesting ways. For example, by stimulating the breeding centre in the brainstem while applying weak currents to the flight centre they suppressed the flight response that would normally occur after this stimulation. They could also induce hybrid behaviours, for example by stimulating the flight and attack centres simultaneously. In this scenario, the chicken would neither attack nor flee but run around with ruffled feathers. However, even this was not a completely new behaviour because it corresponded to a natural reaction to danger. Thus, stimulation of the brain of animals could evoke complex behaviours and modify response tendencies in often dramatic ways, but did not induce behaviours that were outside the animal's natural repertoire.

At about the same time, the Spanish neurophysiologist Jose Delgado set up a programme of brain stimulation work in colonies of cats and monkeys at Yale University. Delgado's aim was to modulate behaviour in realistic, social settings, and he developed devices for the remote control of electrical stimulation to facilitate these experiments.[46] He described the threatening display that could be induced in a cat through anterior hypothalamic stimulation as false or sham rage, but he also demonstrated true rage, directed against another cat or against the experimenter, through stimulation of other, more lateral, sites of the hypothalamus. In colonies of monkeys he studied the interaction of brain stimulation with social hierarchy. One remarkable finding was that the effects of stimulation of a particular nucleus (nucleus posterolateralis) of the thalamus depended on social rank. Delgado placed the same animal in different groups, where it had a high or low status. When it was high up in the group's hierarchy, stimulation would induce it to attack other animals of the group, whereas it only induced non-specific activity (such as running across the cage) when the monkey ranked low in the hierarchy of the respective group. This observation can be interpreted in different ways. The animal's final behaviour may have been under the influence of two competing control processes, the activating thalamic stimulation and a (perhaps cortical) inhibitory control centre that assessed the likely adverse outcome of an attack when the animal was of low rank. Alternatively, brain stimulation may not completely determine the behavioural programme, but only trigger programmes that are within an animal's repertoire in a particular situation. There is experimental evidence to support both explanations.

In favour of the idea of competing control processes, Delgado found that in some cases where he stimulated motor control centres the resulting action did indeed correspond to the algebraic summation of the electrical stimulation and the voluntary or spontaneous motor programme. For example, if the effects of electrical stimulation and the animal's goal-directed behaviour were in the same direction, the animal would produce an overly strong motor response and overshoot its target. Conversely, other experiments favoured the explanation that electrical stimulation could only induce behaviours that were within an animal's natural repertoire at that moment in time. For example, a particular electrical stimulation induced flexion of the right forepaw in a cat, but not when it was in the middle of a jump. However, in Delgado's experiments it was always possible for the experimenter to overrule the natural action tendencies by increasing the strength of the electrical stimulation. But even Delgado did not claim to induce completely new behaviours, just to be able to stop an animal's natural, instinctive reaction.

Delgado also reported inhibitory effects on an animal's hierarchical behaviour. For example, the leading monkey of a group, the so-called alpha animal, has a natural tendency to attack other animals, which Delgado suppressed with stimulation of the caudate nucleus. His most dramatic demonstration of the suppression of instinctive behaviour was perhaps the control of a charging bull that was stopped by electrical stimulation of the caudate nucleus when he was at full throttle in the arena (Figure 2.4). However, Delgado himself acknowledged that part of this effect was caused by the basic motor effects of the stimulation, which forced the bull to turn to one side. Whether, as claimed by Delgado, the stimulation also inhibited the bull's aggressive drive, is impossible to say in the case of an animal whose mental states we can only infer from its behaviour.

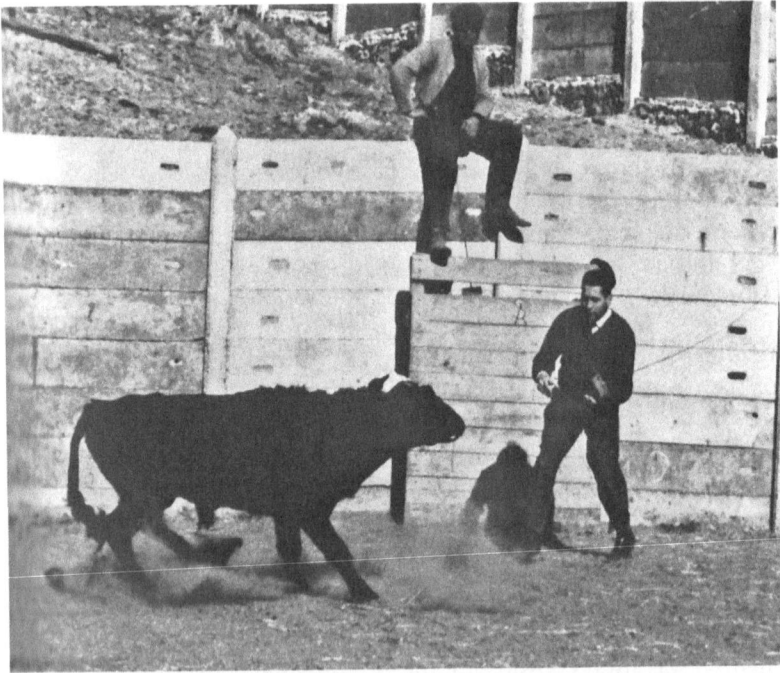

Figure 2.4   Delgado stopping a charging bull by means of a radiotransmitter that controls an electrode in the bull's caudate nucleus (figure 24 from Delgado[46] with kind permission of Caroline Delgado)

Caroline Delgado's account of her late husband's work

Delgado implanted electrodes in patients in 1952, and also Bickford at the Mayo Clinic – Delgado studied colonies of cats, rhesus monkeys, gibbons, chimps and the brave bulls – seeking to demonstrate that aggression can be diminished/blocked in many species. In patients he evoked happy states and suppressed intractable pain. The Chemitrodes were a great innovation, to study electrical and chemical activity in the brain simultaneously. He was the first to invent methods for radio stimulation in free subjects. The colony of gibbons on Hall's Island in Bermuda was amazing. He was the first to do brain to computer to brain stimulation (in chimps so that a normal pattern of electrical activity was sent to the computer where it activated another brain center in the chimp which inhibited the first activity – this was a plan to recognize and block epileptic attacks before they started acting in the brain). Remember, no one was studying groups of animals able to live together in cages or in freedom on an island … repetitive studies were more significant than previous studies during brain operations.

Delgado himself noted the following limitations of his procedure: it was often difficult to predict the behavioural effects of the stimulation of a particular region because the same brain region was responsible for different functions (functional pleiotropy); only a limited set of behaviours was inducible (functional monotony); and one had to rely on skills already learnt by an animal. He thought that brain stimulation could not create a new personality but only enhance or inhibit elements of existing personality:

> We can influence emotional reactivity and perhaps make a patient more aggressive or amorous, but in each case the details of behavioural expression are related to an individual history which cannot be created by ESB.[46]

Regardless of these limitations, relatively simple brain stimulation could induce or suppress complex natural behaviours in Delgado's experiments. This might be particularly relevant if one wanted to re-programme the behaviour of patients who do not conform to societal norms. The ethics of such applications of brain stimulation will be discussed below (Chapter 4). First, we need to explore whether electrical stimulation can really alter human personality?

Deep brain stimulation in humans

The development of stereotactic techniques in the 1940s and 1950s allowed neurosurgeons to access specific structures, for example the hypothalamus, thalamus or amygdala, with high precision by inserting an electrode through a small burr hole in the skull, without the need to perform an open operation on the brain.

These early stereotactic procedures were guided by simple X-ray images of the skull that often involved cumbersome procedures for delineating the cerebral ventricles. The electrode position was standardised through frames mounted on the skull, which provided a coordinate system for the movement of the electrodes at the right angle and distance (Figure 2.5). This is still essentially the procedure used today for Deep Brain Stimulation (DBS) for conditions such as Parkinson's disease, except that the simple X-ray has been replaced by CT (computed tomography) or MRI (magnetic resonance imaging) scans that actually show the tissue of the brain as well, and allow the surgeon to assess whether the electrode is in the right place.

Unlike Penfield's cortical mapping studies, the subcortical stimulation experiments of the 1940s–1960s were not a by-product of a therapeutic procedure (temporal lobe surgery for epilepsy, in Penfield's case), but were intended to be therapeutic interventions in their own right. Several psychiatrists set up such invasive treatment programmes, mainly for schizophrenia but also for a range of other mental or behavioural conditions. The best known of these programmes is that of Dr Robert

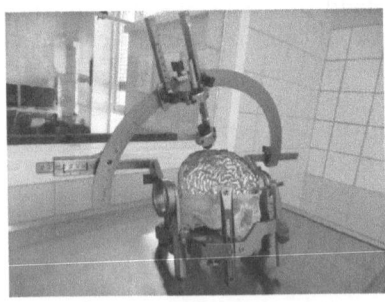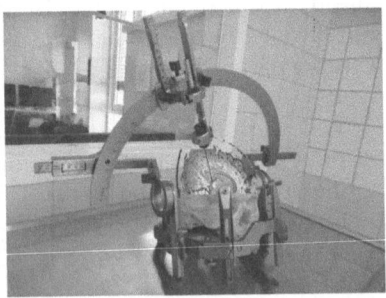

Figure 2.5 Stereotactic apparatus

Note: The left panel shows a stereotactic frame and the surface of the brain (in reality this would be covered by the skull into which only a small burrhole or twist-drill hole is made). The right panel shows a virtual cut in the sagittal plane to illustrate the final electrode position in the basal ganglia region. Photographs courtesy of Professor Volker Arnd Coenen, Freiburg University, Germany..

Heath, the long-term head of the Department of Psychiatry at Tulane University in New Orleans. Heath was dissatisfied with the outcomes and rather crude methodology of frontal lobotomies, then a common surgical treatment for schizophrenia in American asylums (see Section 2.9). He had been a member of one of the programmes to evaluate surgical procedures for mental disorders and he concluded that:

> Cortical ablation of parts of the frontal lobe (lobotomy and topectomy) had produced only minor changes in emotion, perception, and memory of psychotic schizophrenia patients. They continued to have profound emotional impairment, disordered thinking (delusions), and sensory disturbances (hallucinations). The results suggested that the frontal cortex influenced the neural mechanism for emotion, but was not integral to it. On the other hand, ablation or stimulation of certain subcortical sites of animals so profoundly altered emotional behaviour as to suggest that the neural network for emotion was largely subcortical.[47]

Heath wanted to explore the effects of stimulation of specific subcortical structures on patients with schizophrenia. His first target was the septal area, which is a link between the hypothalamus and the limbic system. In total 66 patients had electrodes inserted into this region, and some of them also had miniature cannulas implanted to allow for the delivery of drugs to specific brain sites. Heath reported that this programme only included patients who had failed to respond to all other available treatments and had provided informed consent. Patients with schizophrenia were his largest group, but Heath also included a few patients with chronic, intractable pain. His rationale was that if septal stimulation produced pleasure, and if pleasure was the opposite of pain (which not all emotion researchers would agree with), stimulation of this region should also improve pain. This stimulation did indeed induce pleasurable feelings in many patients. Other areas where stimulation could induce pleasure were the lateral amygdala and a part of the midbrain called the interpeduncular nucleus. The clinicians also had the impression that patients became livelier and more aware of their surroundings. The pleasurable experience was rather undirected and could be attached to whatever stimulus or activity was at hand. Subcortical stimulation could make them enjoy their lunch more or become interested in an erotic movie, depending on the circumstances in which it was delivered, but the internal stimulus did not induce sexual arousal when the external stimulus (the movie) was missing. These results match those of Delgado's monkey experiments, where the reinforcing effects of deep brain stimulation were strongest when it was compatible with the natural tendencies of the animal.

Self-stimulation

An even more direct path to studying the emotional states induced by brain stimulation was opened up when the American physiologist James Olds introduced electrical self-stimulation into animal behaviour research.[10, 48–50] This research programme was triggered by a serendipitous observation he made in 1953 when working in Hebb's laboratory at McGill University in Montreal. He applied electrical stimulation to the region around the anterior commissure, a small white matter bridge between the hemispheres, and found that rats stimulated in this region "would come back for more".[43] Initially, the stimulator was controlled by the experimenter and stimulation was only available in a certain part of the cage, which became the animal's preferred place. Olds then went on to modify a Skinner box so that animals could control the stimulation by pushing or releasing a lever.[43] He replaced the mechanism whereby food would be released upon lever presses with one where the lever could trigger a brief high frequency electrical stimulation delivered through an electrode that had been implanted into the rat's brain.

When given the opportunity to self-stimulate in this way rats would do so, and often with a high degree of persistence. Olds started a large-scale programme where he implanted electrodes into many different areas of the rat brain and found that he could elicit self-stimulation in about a third of the rat brain, a much higher proportion than he had expected. The rats self-stimulated without any additional training, which suggested that for them the electrical stimulus was a primary, or natural, reward, similar to food or sex. However, the results from the Skinner box experiments allowed for the alternative explanation that brain stimulation just induced the rats to engage in compulsive lever pressing. Olds ruled out this possibility by showing that the opportunity to self-stimulate served as a reward in many experimental settings and that he could use it to train rats to navigate a complex maze just as well as if he was using food rewards.[48] He also identified areas where animals would work to avoid or stop stimulation. Olds reckoned that these areas with aversive effects of stimulation occupied only about 5% of the rat's brain. Stimulation in some areas could even be both rewarding and aversive, depending on the stimulation strength.

Olds travelled through the whole brain with his stimulation electrodes, implanting great numbers of rats (each rat only received electrodes in a single or very few brain sites). One of the main areas with rewarding properties was the medial forebrain bundle (MFB). This collection of nerve fibres runs through the septal area and connects three parts of the brain that are crucial for the control of behaviour and bodily functions, the hypothalamus, limbic system and areas controlling motivation in the basal ganglia and midbrain. Stimulation of many other areas in the midbrain, basal ganglia, hypothalamus and cortex was also rewarding. The strongest effects, measured by the frequency with which rats would press the lever, were obtained in the tegmentum area of the midbrain. With electrodes implanted in this area, rats would press the lever up to 7,000 times per hour. In cortical areas rates were lower, only up to 200 times per hour. Another difference between cortical and hypothalamic or midbrain stimulation was that, when the electrodes were placed in cortical areas such as the cingulate gyrus, the self-stimulation period was always limited. Conversely, when electrodes were placed in the hypothalamus, self-stimulation could go on to the level of exhaustion, in some cases for over 24 hours. In some areas, the stimulation effects seemed to depend on the elicitation of specific brain wave patterns, spike-wave complexes that are also a hallmark of epileptic seizures. For example, self-stimulation of the medial forebrain bundle could evoke spike-wave complexes in the septal nuclei during the period when self-stimulation was particularly effective.[51]

In fact, some research reports suggested that animals took the stimulation to a point where they induced seizures in themselves, particularly when the self-stimulation electrodes were placed in the hippocampus. Although it may sound surprising that seizures would be pleasurable, there is clinical evidence from children with certain types of epilepsy who had the habit of inducing seizures in themselves. They did this by waving their hands in front of their eyes and thus inducing a light flicker, which can trigger seizures. Some of these children reported the seizures to be pleasurable (although unpleasant experiences, such as fear, are generally more common during seizures).

The prospect of self-stimulation of the hypothalamus and midbrain areas proved to be a very strong reinforcer, stronger even than food in hungry rats, although the animals never completely stopped eating. Rats would even run over an electrified grid to reach the lever for self-stimulation. Although they also crossed the grid for food, the electrical current in the grid that they would tolerate when the offered reward was self-stimulation was twice as high as that tolerated for food. Olds inferred from this observation that the electrical stimulation was even more rewarding than food, which is commonly thought to be the strongest natural reward for hungry rodents.

The relationship between self-stimulation and other primary rewards was interesting. The hypothalamus is also a main area for the control of feeding behaviour, and some of the rewarding areas also produced behaviours related to food consumption or sexual behaviour, for example ejaculations,[52] when stimulated. Further evidence that the stimulation was tapping into some of the circuits for natural rewards came from the observation that hungry rats were keener to train for self-stimulation than sated animals.

Did Olds's experimental animals become addicted to this self-stimulation? The answer to this question depends on one's definition of addiction. In today's clinical definition, addiction comprises a set of behaviours and attitudes that go beyond mere excessive use, for example escalation of the dose over time, continuation of drug use in the face of adverse consequences, preference for the drug over other choices and an increasingly narrow focus of interest on the drug of abuse.[53] Obviously, there are limitations to modelling these criteria in animals, which were developed to describe human drug addiction. However, the rats in the self-stimulation experiments showed at least some of the behaviours characteristic of addiction: they stimulated until exhaustion when the drug (in this case the electrical current) was available; they went to the place where stimulation was delivered, even if this entailed punishment by electric shock to their limbs; and they neglected food intake, although not completely. They also gradually increased the rate of stimulation, which is akin to another characteristic feature of human addiction, the development of tolerance, which implies that ever-increasing doses of the pharmacological or physical stimulus are needed to obtain the desired psychological effect.

Similar behaviours were observed in later studies in which addictive drugs, for example cocaine, amphetamine, nicotine or heroin, were injected into an animal's blood stream or directly into the brain. Animals preferred to go to places in the cage where these drugs were available and pressed pedals for self-administration, similar to the electrical self-stimulation experiments. Some, but by no means all, animals also showed features of addiction to these substances, as measured by the preference for the drug over food, dose escalation and willingness to take risks to obtain the drug. Only a small minority of rats in cocaine self-administration experiments showed a total loss of control over the drug intake, such that they were prepared to take excessive risks or neglect all other choices. The observation that only a relatively small proportion of rats, approximately 10%, were potential cocaine addicts is interesting for public health efforts to curb drug addiction in humans, for which it would be helpful if we could identify the factors that make individuals vulnerable or resilient to addiction.[53] It also suggests that electrical self-stimulation is a more universal reward than drugs, because the proportion of animals that became hooked on the electrical current was generally higher than those who became addicted in drug self-administration experiments.

The comparison between self-stimulation with electrical current or with drugs also allowed researchers to isolate the neural systems responsible for their rewarding properties. The dopaminergic pathway from the ventral tegmental area in the midbrain to the nucleus accumbens in the basal ganglia, which consists of nerve cells that release the neurotransmitter dopamine, seems to play a prominent role.[54] Olds had observed in the late 1950s that he could block electrical self-stimulation behaviour by treating his animals with the neuroleptic drug chlorpromazine. Although he did know that this drug was effective in treating psychosis, his finding predated the discovery of its main chemical mechanism, blockage of dopamine receptors. Later studies indeed confirmed his observation that dopamine blockers, such as antipsychotic drugs, attenuated the animal's responses to electrical stimulation. Higher currents were required to induce the same rate of lever presses in animals treated with antipsychotics. Conversely, animals treated with amphetamine, a drug that promotes the release of dopamine (see Figure 2.2), put in the same amount of work for much smaller amounts of electrical stimulation.[55]

These findings indicate that the rewarding effect of electrical self-stimulation operates through dopaminergic pathways. They were supported by studies with direct self-administration of dopaminergic drugs, such as amphetamine, where animals consistently preferred conditions where the drug was applied directly into the nucleus accumbens.[54, 56] Even the self-administration of drugs from other classes, for example heroin and other opioids, seems to obtain its rewarding properties from the activation of dopaminergic pathways.[5, 54] These close links between the neural pathways of electrical (self-)stimulation and drugs of abuse are clinically important today for the evaluation of the risks and benefits of DBS. As we will see in Section 2.11, psychiatric patients receiving DBS often suffer a relapse when the stimulator is switched off (or when the battery is empty). This might indicate that the DBS treatment actually worked very well and is needed for symptom control. Alternatively, it might indicate that patients become addicted to DBS after the many months or years of stimulation and that any discontinuation produces unpleasant withdrawal symptoms. DBS can only be called a reversible procedure if the latter scenario is unlikely and risk of addiction to DBS is low. We will come back to this question in Chapter 4.

Olds and the other pioneers of self-stimulation research in animals could only infer the pleasurable experience associated with the electrical stimulation from its reinforcing properties and the animal's stimulus-seeking behaviour. However, the opportunity soon arose to compare these results with direct self-reports that could be obtained from humans. In the context of their work on therapeutic DBS, Heath's group developed a device for self-stimulation in humans, which was used by a number of patients who had electrodes implanted into different subcortical sites. The patients could not only control when and for how long they were stimulated, but also at which of the implanted sites. As expected on the basis of Olds's self-stimulation experiments in animals, the hypothalamic regions were the favourites, followed by the periaqueductal grey matter of the midbrain, which contains opioid-sensitive neurons, and the lateral amygdala. With hypothalamic self-stimulation patients felt euphoric, while self-stimulation of other areas, notably the septal region, allowed them to suppress pain. Heath reports the anecdote that one of the patients was so pleased with the experience that she even asked to get married to the experimenter.

Aversive experiences

Stimulation of some deep brain areas had the opposite effect. Rather than evoking pleasant experiences it made patients fearful, angry and sometimes even violent.[47] These areas included the tegmentum area of the midbrain, hypothalamus, medial amygdala (the lateral amygdala was associated with positive experiences) and the hippocampus. One of Heath's patients became "murderously rageful" and threatened to kill the physician standing next to him during the stimulation. "I felt like a gorilla and wanted to kill", he later said about his state. However, even in this case, the brain stimulation did not induce a completely novel, out of character state in the stimulated person. According to Heath, this patient reported that he had felt a similar rage against his mother during his adolescent years.

Brain sites where stimulation evoked pleasant or aversive experiences were often in close proximity, for example in the midbrain. It was also sometimes difficult to keep the stimulation focal enough to induce only the desired response. For example, although stimulation of the lateral amygdala was generally experienced as pleasant, if the current applied to this region was too strong it could also induce rage, possibly because stimulation seeped through to the medial amygdala. Moreover, the stimulation results in humans were not always congruent with those from animals, which perhaps is not very surprising considering the differences between the human and rat brain even in these evolutionarily old structures. Whereas Olds had consistently elicited pleasurable responses from a stimulation of the medial forebrain bundle, Heath only obtained aversive responses to stimulation of analogous regions in the rostral hypothalamus. His patients became anxious and developed signs of a panic attack.[57] He explained that his stimulation may not have been focused enough on targeting positive emotion pathways. Again, this is an important issue for any clinical application of DBS, particularly in psychiatry.

Brain stimulation – lasting effects?

One of the main challenges for therapeutic brain stimulation was – and still is – to produce effects that lasted beyond the acute stimulation protocol. As discussed by Valenstein,[44] the idea championed by Heath and Delgado was that the pleasurable experience in itself could be therapeutic and trigger subsequent positive processes, acting as a kind of emotion pacemaker. This idea is not radically different from some psychotherapeutic concepts, where the time-limited induction of a specific mental state through mental imagery is supposed to facilitate the therapeutic process. In addition, both Heath and Delgado developed methods for long-term electrical stimulation through indwelling electrodes and for local delivery of specific doses of neurotransmitters or other drugs through implanted cannulae. Heath reported that he obtained effects with local acetylcholine administration similar to those from electrical stimulation: pleasure, including orgasms in the septal region; rage and fear in the hippocampus.

Did brain stimulation help patients with schizophrenia?

What then is the evidence that these early DBS programmes actually improved patient symptoms or enhanced their quality of life, for example, by making it possible to discharge them from long-term institutional care? Perhaps to expect such improvements was always against the odds if we side with Valenstein's polemic that: "The belief that anyone could adjust in this world if a spontaneous orgasm followed by a detached mental calmness was programmed in at 10, 2, and 6 o'clock seems ludicrous."[44]

The evaluation of treatment programmes in the 1950s and 1960s did not follow the same principles as psychiatric trials today, which use control or placebo interventions wherever possible and incorporate assessments with standardised rating scales where the assessor is blind to the type of intervention. It is therefore difficult to assess just how clinically useful this generation of brain stimulation programmes for mental disorders was. It seems, though, that for all their spectacular immediate effects on mental states and behaviour, these brain stimulation protocols did not produce lasting therapeutic benefits in the majority of psychiatric patients, even when Heath and his colleagues developed electrodes that could remain in place and deliver stimulation over several months. Furthermore, many of their patients with chronic schizophrenia suffered from the characteristic symptoms of anhedonia (inability to experience joy) and apathy (lack of drive), which today's psychiatrists call negative symptoms, and these patients showed less dramatic immediate effects of the stimulation than those with epilepsy or chronic pain. Although Heath had been optimistic about the outcome for his first series of 20 patients with schizophrenia, it was not possible to control for other factors that may have contributed to the improvement seen in some of the patients, such as increased attention given to patients enrolled in experimental treatment programmes in a large mental hospital setting. Heath himself later abandoned deep brain stimulation in schizophrenia and pursued it only in patients with neurological disorders or chronic pain.

Unlike the huge wave of lobotomies, which we will encounter later in this chapter (Section 2.9), subcortical brain stimulation for psychiatric disorders never spread beyond specialised academic centres. However, like lobotomy, its further development was virtually abandoned when the antipsychotic drugs that appeared in the mid-1950s offered a non-invasive way of controlling a patient's symptoms and, in many cases, improving their quality of life. Reviewing the evidence in 1973, Valenstein concluded:

> Although the phenomenon of evoked mood and mental status changes that last beyond the stimulation has been sufficiently documented that it can happen, there is no convincing evidence that these changes have ever contributed significantly to any cures.[44]

2.4 The shaking palsy

Yet there is one brain disorder where most physicians would agree that deep brain stimulation has contributed to the alleviation of suffering, Parkinson's disease. This disease was first described in 1817, when the English apothecary James Parkinson (1755–1824) published a small book entitled *An Essay on the Shaking Palsy*. He had observed a few patients with an unusual "tremulous motion", partly in his practice and partly during casual encounters in the streets of London. This first case was:

> a man rather more than fifty years of age, who had industriously followed the business of a gardener, leading a life of remarkable temperance and sobriety. The commencement of the malady was first manifested by a slight trembling of the left hand and arm, a circumstance which he was disposed to attribute to his having been engaged for several days in a kind of employment requiring considerable exertion of that limb.

However, it turned out that the trembling was not caused by the exertion but became rather more severe over time. It made it almost impossible for the patients to write or eat or drink without help. Other characteristic features that Parkinson observed were "a propensity to bend the trunk forwards, and to pass from a walking to a running pace". Patients had to take smaller and faster steps and found it difficult both to start and to stop walking. Although the disease progressed slowly, at some point it severely disrupted patient's lives, affecting their sleep and bowel functions. Yet "the senses and intellects" remained "uninjured."

Parkinson provided very astute observations of the early presentation and progression of several cases of this classic movement disorder, which was named in his honour by the great French neurologist Jean-Martin Charcot (1825–1893). Parkinson was right about the early symptoms and had correctly described the one-sided tremor and shuffling gait, as well as the debilitating balance problems. He had also noted that vegetative functions, such as sleep or bowel motions, were affected at later stages. However, he was too optimistic about the "uninjured intellects". We know today that about 50% of patients with Parkinson's disease go on to suffer cognitive impairment, or even dementia, as a consequence of the illness.

Parkinson was also wrong about the cause; he located it in the spinal cord, whereas today we know that it is the loss of cells producing the neurotransmitter dopamine in the midbrain that causes the motor symptoms of Parkinson's disease. The area that is primarily affected is called substantia nigra, or black substance, because dopaminergic neurons contain high levels of the black pigment melanin. The first motor symptoms start when the substantia nigra loses 60% of its dopaminergic neurons. The substantia nigra is embedded in a network of nuclei, or basal ganglia, accumulations of nerve cells that are buried in the depths of the brain and control the fine tuning of movements.

As explained in the circuit diagram of Figure 2.6, the loss of input from the substantia nigra changes the balance of excitatory and inhibitory connections between the basal ganglia and leads to a net decrease in impulses sent from the thalamus to the cortex. This could explain the often severe difficulty in initiating movement, which is a key function of cortical motor regions, and the general slowing of motor behaviour. Other disorders of the basal ganglia, where the changes go in the opposite direction and lead to increased output, are characterised by uncontrolled excessive movements. One of these hyperkinetic diseases is Huntington's disease, an inherited neurodegenerative disorder starting in the striatum and characterised by chorea, irregular jerky movements of the limbs and trunk.

Recent work on PD has shown that other areas further down in the brainstem may be affected even earlier than the dopamine-producing midbrain cells, and that several other neurotransmitters (serotonin, noradrenalin, acetylcholine) are depleted as well. However, we know that dopamine is the key player because if patients are treated with analogues of dopamine they improve dramatically. With these drugs many patients can lead relatively unimpaired lives over many years and continue to work and pursue their hobbies. Alyssa Johnson, a 43-year old Parkinson's sufferer, even completed the Boston marathon in a very respectable six hours. This and other sporting achievements by PD patients are documented on the website of the Michael Fox Foundation (https://www.michaeljfox.org). The main drugs used for Parkinson's are levodopa, which is a chemical precursor of dopamine that can be converted into dopamine in the brain, and a group of dopamine agonist drugs, which mimic the effects of dopamine on brain cells. Although these drugs work well for the classic triad of Parkinson's symptoms (tremor, rigidity and slowness to move), they are generally only effective for a few hours after administration – called the "on" period – and patients have to develop strategies to cope with the periods when the drug's effects wear off – the so-called "off" periods. The overall dose of dopaminergic drugs that can be administered is limited by the numerous side effects, which include other motor problems (dyskinesias) and personality changes, which, in

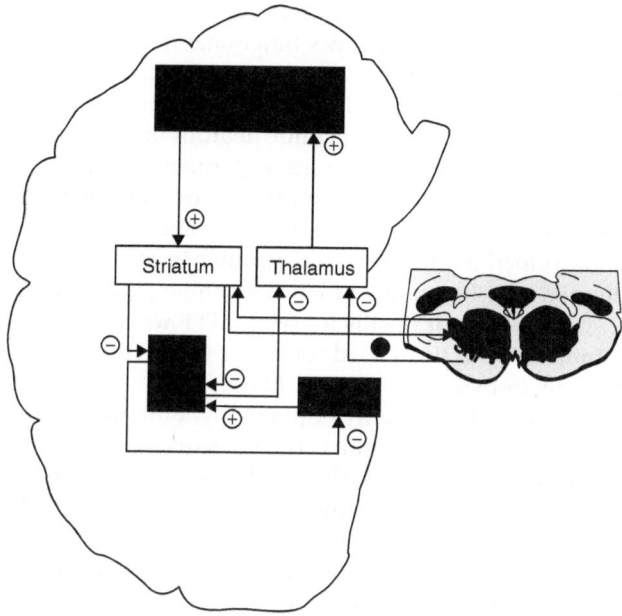

Figure 2.6   Circuit schema of Parkinson's disease (PD) pathophysiology

Note: The direct and indirect pathways of the basal ganglia are important for the understanding of Parkinson's disease. The basal ganglia (striatum: putamen and caudate nucleus; globus pallidus, external and internal parts [GPe, GPi], subthalamic nucleus [STN] and thalamus) form an important loop for motor control (in addition to other sensory and homoeostatic functions not shown here). The striatum is the main input station of the basal ganglia and receives excitatory (glutamatergic) input from motor cortex. The main output station is the (ventrolateral/ventral anterior) thalamus, which sends excitatory projections to (pre-)motor cortex. The striatum regulates the thalamic motor nuclei through a direct (through the GPi) and an indirect (through GPe, STN and GPi) loop and further loops through the substantia nigra, pars reticulata (SNr). The striatal function is modulated by dopaminergic input from the substantia nigra, pars compacta (SNc), which is disrupted in Parkinson's disease. From Linden, *The Biology of Psychological Disorders*.[5]

some patients, can even amount to problem gambling, overspending, increased sex drive and aggression. These side effects become worse over the years. This was the reason for exploring other treatment avenues, based not on drugs but on direct electrical modulation of the brain.

2.5   DBS and Parkinson's disease

After DBS's initial failure in psychiatry the attention of functional neurosurgeons using it turned to neurological disorders, particularly those affecting the movement circuits of the basal ganglia. PD has become the main target for today's functional neurosurgeons because its biology is relatively well known and can be modelled in animals, and because the initial clinical results were very promising. Although the primary reason for the loss of dopamine neurons in the substantia nigra in PD is still undiscovered, there are experimental ways of inducing similar processes through the use of drugs. This happened accidentally when students tried to synthesise the substance MPPP (1-Methyl-4-phenyl-4-oxypiperidine), which was popular in the 1970s and 1980s as an alternative to heroin because it has similar psychological effects. One particular danger of the illicit use of MPPP was that it could easily be contaminated with the related substance MPTP (1-Methyl-4-phenyl-1,2,3,6-tetrahydropyridine). In the brain, MPTP is converted to a substance called MPP+ (1-Methyl-4-phenylpyridinium), which destroys the dopamine-producing neurons. The students came to the attention of American neurologists because they developed symptons of PD at a very young age, and ultimately the link to the MPTP consumption was discovered. These doctors had thus discovered the first drug-induced model of Parkinson's disease. Because the same effects of dopamine loss and motor symptoms can also be seen in monkeys, it allowed researchers to study new therapies in monkeys who had been exposed to MPTP. In monkeys, the effects of the loss of dopamine neurons in the substantia nigra, or other parts of the basal ganglia, could be studied in much more detail than in humans by measuring the electrical activity directly with implanted electrodes. One of the striking findings was that the nerve cells in the basal ganglia did not simply fire less in the Parkinson's monkeys, but that some areas were actually overactive. One of these areas was the subthalamic nucleus. The various parts of the basal ganglia send inhibitory and excitatory projections to each other, and this system is normally in a delicate balance (Figure 2.6). The loss of dopamine neurons results in failure to inhibit the subthalamic nucleus, which then fires excessively. This in turn inhibits another deep structure, the thalamus, which is a major gateway to the motor cortex. The net result is lack of input into the areas involved in voluntary motor control, which manifests itself in the difficulty with movement initiation that is so typical of Parkinson's patients.

This finding of overactivity in parts of the basal ganglia opened up an exciting treatment possibility. The researchers soon realised that trying to replace the lost dopamine neurons would be a major challenge. The necessary tools for cellular and molecular biology simply were not available in the 1980s, and even today, with stem cell technology at their fingertips, Parkinson's researchers are just beginning to create functioning dopaminergic neurons that can be implanted into patients' brains. Thus, the rationale of the pioneers of DBS for PD was that one might restore the balance of the motor control loops by deactivating the subthalamic nucleus. The initial approach, reported in 1990 in the journal *Science*, was to destroy this area in MPTP monkeys, which did in fact lead to the disappearance of Parkinson's symptoms.[58]

This approach to Parkinson's was not entirely new. For decades surgeons had tried to improve the symptoms of advanced Parkinson's by inserting heat probes into specific parts of the basal ganglia and destroying them.[59] The main problem with this approach was that it only worked for some patients and some symptoms. The data coming out of the monkey model pointed to new target areas, and made neurologists hopeful that silencing the subthalamic nucleus and other overactive structures might improve the plight of large numbers of patients for whom drugs had ceased to work. The new approach was not to produce irreversible lesions in these areas, but to modulate their activity with deep brain stimulation. This procedure consists of inserting an electrode into the target area, for example the subthalamic nucleus, and connecting it to a long-life battery that is placed in a pouch under the skin of the chest, similar to a cardiac pacemaker. The electrode can then stimulate the targeted area over many years, and the physician can control the frequency by changing the settings on the pacemaker. This approach is attractive because settings, such as stimulation intensity (current strength, voltage and pulse width) and frequency, can be changed according to the clinical response, whereas lesions are irreversible.

By stimulating the subthalamic nucleus at high frequencies (over 100 Hz) it is possible to obtain stunning and immediate effects on patient movements. For example, patients who were stuck in a chair are able to lift themselves up and move freely after the stimulator is switched on. Tremors are suppressed and rigid muscles relax again. Balance problems and difficulties with speaking improve less by comparison, or can even become worse in some cases.[60] Symptoms improve most on the side contralateral to the stimulation because most of motor control in the brain is crossed (and thus the left side of the brain controls the muscles on the right side of the body and vice versa). This led to procedures where electrodes were implanted into the subthalamic nuclei on both sides of the brain (bilateral stimulation), which produced even better effects [61, 62] (but also higher risk of surgical and cognitive side effects).

The basic neurophysiological effects of DBS are multi-faceted and can entail both inhibition and excitation of the stimulated and downstream regions. For example, both ipsilateral and contralateral DBS of the subthalamic nucleus at high frequencies (>100 Hz) can reduce the firing rate of neurons in this region from around 19 Hz (19 action potentials per second) to around 8 Hz.[63] Similar effects can be observed for the local field potential, a measure that integrates across thousands of neurons from a brain area and is, in many respects, similar to the EEG (except that it has a much higher spatial resolution and does not suffer from attenuation through transmission through brain and skull because it is recorded directly from the area of interest – obviously such recordings are only possible when electrodes are inserted during medically necessary surgical procedures). The beta frequency band (12 Hz–30 Hz) in particular shows marked attenuation both immediately and months after the insertion of the DBS electrode.[64] Such suppression of neuronal activity may explain why high frequency DBS has similar clinical effects to lesions in the same area (whereas stimulation of the basal ganglia with frequencies under 25 Hz can induce symptoms such as tremor). A simple model of the effects of high frequency DBS on the subthalamic nucleus (STN) would then posit that this stimulation inhibits the STN, leading to a reduction of activity in its projection area in the internal globus pallidus (GPi). Because the projections of the GPi to the thalamus are inhibitory, the suppression of GPi firing would actually lead to an increase of thalamic activity and consequently enhanced activation of cortical motor areas, which would lead to improved motor control (Figure 2.6).

Yet the reality is probably more complex. Studies in monkey models of PD with stimulation in the STN and recordings in the GPi have actually shown that activity in the GPi was increased. It is still unclear why suppression of the STN would lead to such a paradoxical increase in GPi activity when STN projections to the GPi are generally thought to be excitatory. However, this observation points to alternative accounts of the clinical benefits of DBS in PD. It is important to consider that the neurophysiological effects of DBS can be observed in distances of several millimetres. Most basal ganglia nuclei extend over only a few millimetres and thus DBS is likely to affect other areas or fibre tracts passing through them. This could lead to stimulation of the substantia nigra and thus to additional dopamine release or to the activation of compensatory motor circuits.[63] It is also worth remembering that similar clinical effects can be obtained by DBS in several brain areas, not just the STN, but also GPi, GPe, the pedunculopontine nucleus in the brainstem and possibly even the motor cortex itself.[63] Such a model of generic motor pathway activation would provide a rationale for exploring other means of activating compensatory pathways, for example through neurofeedback, which will be discussed in Chapter 3.

In the UK, the whole DBS procedure, including assessments, surgery, battery pack and electrode and inpatient stay, costs about £30,000. It is estimated that 60,000 PD patients worldwide have been treated with DBS. Yet, this is only about 1% of the estimated 6 million people worldwide who suffer from PD. Patients who undergo surgery for DBS have, on average, been diagnosed 14 years earlier. This relatively long delay from initial diagnosis to consideration for surgery is interesting because it indicates that for many patients modern drug treatment works well for long periods of time, and that DBS is still considered to be a treatment of last resort. However, the overall numbers also suggest that only a small proportion of PD patients will actually go on to receive DBS. There are many reasons for this. Surgery for DBS is an invasive procedure with potential complications, such as bleeds or infections in the brain or the development of epileptic fits. Not all patients have the kinds of side effects or difficult-to-treat motor symptoms that would warrant DBS in order to improve symptom control and/or reduce the drug doses. Most importantly, many patients live in countries where DBS is not available on public health systems. At the same time, researchers are exploring whether DBS should actually be employed earlier for improved symptom control. EARLYSTIM, the first trial of DBS in patients in the earlier stages of PD, which included a follow-up over two years, was published in early 2013 with encouraging results.[65, 66] Perhaps most importantly, the patients in the DBS group managed to reduce their dopaminergic medication by about a third, whilst still having slightly better outcomes than the "treatment as usual" group. This is important because some of the medication side effects seem to depend on the overall amount of anti-Parkinson's medication that a patient has taken over their lifetime. Patients who underwent DBS also reported an improved quality of life. However, they also suffered from some surgical side effects, for example infection.

If further trials confirm a clinical benefit of early DBS intervention demand for DBS is likely to increase, and the gap between high-tech treatment in industrialised countries and standard drug treatment (or in some countries for many patients no treatment at all) in most of the rest of the world is likely to widen. Like any age-related disorder, PD, generally regarded as the second most common brain degeneration after Alzheimer's disease, is going to become more prevalent with the worldwide increase in life expectancy. About 1% of over 70-year olds suffer from it and patient numbers are expected to grow especially rapidly in the developing countries of Asia and Latin America. Finding a cure for PD is thus one of the big health challenges of our time. At the moment, nobody really knows how to prevent the degeneration of the dopamine neurons in PD and the attempts to replace them with stem cells, or stimulate them to grow again with so-called growth factors, are in the very early stages of development. In the absence of a cure, the refinement of treatments that allow patients to overcome their symptoms and lead functional and fulfilled lives is therefore paramount. Every patient with PD will require medication for the foreseeable future, and some will continue to benefit from DBS. But might it be possible to harness some of the advances of brain self-regulation techniques to benefit PD patients as well? We will come back to this question when we discuss new neurofeedback-based treatments in neurology and psychiatry in Chapter 3. For now we will turn to other neurological applications for DBS.

2.6   DBS for other movement disorders: tremor and dystonia

Although PD is a relatively common neurodegenerative disorder and its prevalence in ageing populations will continue to increase, it is by no means the most common movement disorder. Approximately ten times as many people, 1% of the population, are affected by a condition called essential tremor, although many of them never see a doctor for their motor problems. Essential tremor (ET) is characterised by a symmetrical shaking of the hands and forearms. This occurs during particular postures, for example when stretching out the hands, or movements, for example moving a cup to the mouth. These types of tremors are called postural or kinetic. Resting tremor, which is a core feature of PD, is much less common in ET than postural or kinetic tremor. Patients often also suffer from head tremor. A decisive feature of classic ET, which distinguishes it for example from PD, is that the problems remain confined to this single symptom, tremor, rather than involving other areas of motor function. Although many patients can cope reasonably well with their tremor, and several effective drugs are available, some patients become severely disabled. DBS of a part of the thalamus, the ventrointermedius nucleus (VIM), has been tried in such patients and, although some reports were very promising, better evidence from controlled studies is still needed to judge its efficacy. The VIM is a neuroanatomically plausible target for the treatment of tremor because it is a relay station between the cerebellum and motor cortex, and diseases of the cerebellum can also give rise to different forms of tremor. As always with DBS the potential neurological improvement has to be weighed against the risk of immediate surgical complications, such as bleeds and longer-term side effects. The potential side effects after thalamic stimulation include neurological disturbances such as dysarthria (articulation problems), balance problems or paraes-thesias (uncomfortable sensations).[67] Care must therefore be taken not to cure one neurological problem by causing several others. Another invasive option is surgical destruction of this part of the thalamus, which has been used in the treatment of various types of tremor since the 1950s. However, this procedure, especially if applied on both sides, has a less favourable side effect profile, and many of the patients oper-ated on developed speech and swallowing problems.

The control of tremor by DBS is often very dramatic. When the high frequency stimulator is switched on, symptoms can disappear suddenly and, equally suddenly, recur when it is switched off again. With other movement problems the effects of DBS can take longer and build up over weeks or months of stimulation (which may also be the case for some of the psychiatric effects as we will discuss below). This is particu-larly true for dystonia, a condition, or rather group of conditions, char-acterised by abnormal postures or repetitive movements. The abnormal posture can affect single body parts (focal dystonia), whole segments of the body (segmental dystonia), or even the entire body (generalised dystonia). Examples of focal dystonia are focal hand dystonia or writer's cramp, a loss of control over precision movements of the hands, or torti-collis, twisted neck. Focal hand dystonia is a special case because the symptoms are mainly brought on by particular motor activities, such as trying to write or play a musical instrument, and it is a well-recognised occupational hazard for professional musicians.

The underlying neural mechanisms of dystonia are poorly understood, although one particular problem seems to be the concurrent activation of opposing muscle groups. In the long run, this can result in rather painful, fixed abnormal postures that can be severely disabling. The causes of dystonia can be as varied as its clinical pictures. Some dystonia syndromes are associated with particular genetic mutations and others arise as a consequence of other illnesses or of treatment with antipsy-chotic drugs, but in many cases the cause is unknown.

Most cases of dystonia are difficult to treat with medication. The more focal forms often respond well to local injections of botulinum toxin (Botox), which paralyses muscle activity in the injected area, but this is generally not an option for segmental or generalised dystonia. DBS is an option for patients with disabling symptoms who have not responded well to other treatments. Although other treatment options need to be exhausted before DBS is considered it is also important not to leave it too late because the fixed contractures that can develop over years are almost impossible to resolve with DBS. The main target of DBS in dystonia is the internal globus pallidus (GPi), which is also one of the main targets in PD. As in PD and ET, the development of DBS has been informed by earlier surgical procedures. Destruction of the GPi led to considerable improvement of dystonia symptoms, but, as in other movement disorders, these surgical procedures have been largely abandoned for DBS because of the more favourable side effect profile of the latter.[68] Why DBS of parts of the basal ganglia motor circuit can have such a profound effect on symptoms of movement disorders, and in many cases restore motor control, is largely unknown, although most current models assume that the externally imposed rhythm of high frequency stimulation overrides some dysfunctional network activity and thus restores normal function. What is particularly interesting about DBS for dystonia is that, in addition to building up over a long time, clinical effects can also outlast stimulation by many hours. This suggests that DBS does not just act as a direct pacemaker for the brain's motor circuits but also reshapes them in a more lasting fashion.

2.7 Phantom limb pain and DBS

We have already encountered the motor homunculus in Section 1.2. The sensory representations of the body parts in the brain are also organised in a sequential fashion, starting with the leg at the top of the primary sensory cortex in the parietal lobe and travelling down to the representation of the face just above the Sylvian fissure, which separates the parietal from the temporal lobe.

The pathways that carry information about heat, pain and touch from the periphery to the brain start in receptor and nerve cells in the skin that transmit information to the spinal cord. The information travels up the spinal cord through different tracts and at some point the nerve fibres cross over to the other side, to end up in the thalamus, which is the main relay station for incoming sensory information. Nerve cells in the thalamus pass the signals from specific body parts on to the corresponding regions in the somatosensory cortex, giving rise to the sensory homunculus.

Pain, although unpleasant, is an extremely important sensation for survival because it generally indicates dangerous environmental influences. We therefore have a very rapid learning mechanism that allows us to avoid painful, and thus presumably dangerous, situations. We seem to share this mechanism with many animals. For example, a host of experiments with rodents have shown that painful electric shocks are a very powerful means to teach them to avoid particular parts of their cage. In humans, these memories for painful events can become deeply entrenched, as everyone who has touched a hot oven as a child can confirm. However, such memories can also go awry, as in the classic example of phantom pain. Many patients who have had a limb amputated, for example after an injury, start to report severe pain in this, now non-existent, limb, the phantom. This problem was recognised by military surgeons several hundred years ago and first formally described in veterans of the Civil War by the famous American neurologist Silas Weir Mitchell (1829–1914). Although patients who have an arm or leg removed complain most commonly of phantom pain it can also occur after breast amputation or the removal of internal organs. What sounds completely paradoxical at first – how can a body part that is not there hurt? – can be explained through faulty connections between pain areas in the brain. Of course, the peripheral pain receptors have disappeared with the limb, but its representation in the brain's homunculus is still there. Missing its regular input from the periphery, the area of central representation of the removed limb may just start generating its own patterns of activity, creating phantom sensations, including pain. Although the techniques that allow researchers to monitor brain activity through the intact skull (called non-invasive techniques) are not yet refined enough to prove that such misdirected firing of cells by the homunculus is causing the phantom pain, some studies have actually shown changes in both the motor and the sensory homunculus after limb amputation. A patient who is tormented by pain in his amputated limb might perhaps wonder whether the operation was not quite radical enough, and whether the surgeon should have removed the relevant parts of the brain as well. This proposition is actually not completely outlandish. Lesions of the thalamus (thalamotomy) have been used for a long time in the treatment of intractable pain, based on the rationale that preventing the sensory information from reaching the cortex should alleviate the pain. This procedure has had some success but has now been superseded by deep brain stimulation.[69]

DBS for chronic pain, like any other invasive treatment, is only considered for patients in whom drug treatment and psychological intervention do not produce satisfactory relief. The main target areas are the ventroposterolateral nucleus of the thalamus and the periaqueductal grey matter, an area involved in pain processing located in the brainstem. The exact reasons why DBS in these areas can be effective for pain relief are not known. One reason may indeed be that the propagation of pain-related signals to the cortex is disrupted through the high frequency electrical stimulation. Another potential mechanism may be that DBS triggers the release of opioids, which are well known for their analgesic (pain killer) effects. Based on the above considerations about dysfunction within the homunculus, one might also consider interfering with the cortical representation directly. Motor cortex stimulation (MCS), which is less invasive than DBS because electrodes can be placed on top of the cortex rather than having to be driven deep into the brain, is indeed another possible technique for pain relief that has been used with some success for phantom limb patients.

Although phantom pain occurs in up to 80% of amputees it is still a relatively rare problem. Other chronic pain syndromes are much more common, for example from cancer or after failed back surgery. These types of pain can also potentially be treated with DBS or MCS if other measures fail, although surgeons and anaesthetists are increasingly placing electrodes further down the pain pathway, over the spinal cord. At the moment DBS for pain has an uncertain future because recent trials have not found strong evidence for its efficacy and ultimately it may be superseded by the less invasive options of MCS and spinal cord stimulation.

2.8   DBS and personality

The observation of long-term effects of DBS on motor and sensory function immediately brings up a potential concern. Might there be other – less desirable – long-term changes. Can DBS alter someone's thoughts and emotions, perhaps even turn someone into a completely different person?

There is no easy answer to this question. The history of brain stimulation studies in both animals and humans, from Hess to Heath and Delgado shows that it is certainly possible to influence, even induce, behaviours with electromagnetic stimulation of the brain. Penfield's studies in the 1950s revealed that electrical stimulation of the brain could do more than induce simple movements (such as thumb twitches) or sensory phenomena (such as light flashes). When stimulating the temporal lobe of patients with epilepsy, Penfield induced complex altered states of consciousness and hallucinations in multiple sensory domains. He could also induce people to remember certain events. Although his purpose was to map out epileptic foci for surgical treatment rather than to influence patient behaviour, it is conceivable that such a technique, with permanent electrode implantation, could influence people's mental lives and behaviour in very profound ways. We saw in Section 2.3 that subcortical stimulation, for example of the amygdala or septal area, can indeed influence people's behaviour, at least in the short term. One of the most radical effects of DBS in humans may have been that observed after right thalamic stimulation in a patient with Tourette's syndrome, a neuropsychiatric condition that will be discussed further in Section 2.11.

> Twelve months postoperatively, the patient was hospitalized because he developed a dissociative response when increasing the amplitude of the right stimulation. Manipulation of the stimulation parameters became his usual practice to better control his tics. An increase in amplitude from 1.5 V (the preset level) to 2.4 V (the maximum level) resulted in the following response. He was anxiously crouching in a corner, covering his face with his hands. He spoke with a childish high-pitched voice and repeatedly insisted that he was not to blame. Sentences were brief and grammatically incorrect. If approached by one of us, he fiercely kicked his feet because he feared being thrown in the basement. When the amplitude of the stimulation was lowered to the preset level, behavior was adequate again. Afterward, he could not tell what had happened and reported to have been overwhelmed by bad childhood memories.[70]

This patient seems to have entered into a different identity, as if the stimulation had taken him back to his childhood. Penfield's temporal lobe stimulation had also evoked some vivid memories from childhood, but it never produced the dramatic affective response observed in this patient after thalamic stimulation. It may indeed be the case that subcortical stimulation can produce more drastic changes in a person's feelings and behaviour than cortical stimulation. Yet, for most people undergoing DBS changes in mental state and personality will be far more subtle.

The experience of the 60,000 patients who have so far received DBS for Parkinson's disease, and the many others who have received it for other movement disorders or chronic pain, can give further answers to the question of how it affects the mind. The majority of patients report a clear improvement in their quality of life, mainly due to improved motor control and mobility. However, some of them experience cognitive problems. Verbal fluency is the most commonly affected function. Although these impairments are rarely dramatic and can improve again over time, it is important to remember that the subthalamic nucleus modulates the input of the thalamus to the frontal cortex, which is not only crucial for motor functions but also for cognition. Yet the exact effect of DBS on these circuits is unknown.[71] For example, the negative effect of verbal fluency seems to arise from the electrode implantation itself rather than the delivery of current through it.

The different effects of subcortical stimulation on cognition, mood, behaviour and motor functions can be explained better if we consider the architecture and connections of the commonest targets of DBS in more detail. The basal ganglia are generally divided into three components: motor; cognitive or associative; and affective, or limbic (Figure 2.7).

The affective section of the basal ganglia has close connections with the limbic system (Figure 2.4) that governs emotion and motivation and comprises the amygdala and hippocampus and the cingulate gyrus, an old (in evolutionary terms) part of the frontal lobe. These affective loops between basal ganglia and limbic system can be affected by DBS

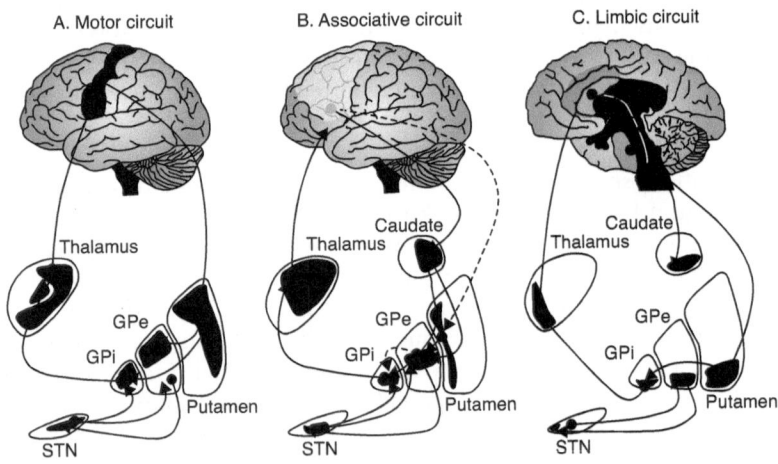

Figure 2.7   The three main circuits of the basal ganglia

Note: (A) The motor circuit connects to the primary (and higher) motor cortices and corresponds to the diagrams drawn in Figure 2.6. (B) The associative circuit supports cognitive functions and connects to the prefrontal cortex, which harbours areas involved in working memory and executive functions. (C) The limbic circuit can also be conceptualised as an extension of the limbic system and is closely connected to the brainstem and cingulate gyrus. Reprinted from [72] and [73] with kind permission of John Wiley and Sons and Elsevier.

as well and this, rather than the effect on motor loops, may explain the most serious adverse effects of longstanding DBS. Mood can change in either direction, resulting in euphoria or lowness, and this can develop into the full psychiatric syndromes of mania and depression. During electrode implantation, even a small displacement of the electrode into a different part of the subthalamic nucleus can induce dramatic changes in behaviour. For example the difference between motor effects and euphoria could be a mere couple of millimetres.[74] Similar to the experience of the early subcortical stimulation studies by Heath and others, the mental states induced by a slight displacement of the stimulation electrodes are not completely out of character but seem to correspond to the patient's pre-formed range of emotional and behavioural responses.

This observation is also clinically important because patients with a previous history of depression and suicide attempts are more likely to become suicidal under DBS. It has been recognised that the severe mood changes that can be produced with DBS, in conjunction with heightened impulsivity, can result in attempted and even completed suicide. One large follow-up study on 5,000 patients found that about 0.5% of patients committed suicide at some point after DBS surgery. Not all of them were necessarily caused by the DBS but the rates were higher than expected in the population, even accounting for the fact that they were sufferers of Parkinson's disease.

DBS of the subthalamic nucleus and other relay stations of the basal ganglia can thus lead to altered mood and personality, with severe behavioural consequences in a small number of cases. Considering the improvement in the quality of life in the majority of cases, this risk may be acceptable, but clinicians are working hard to identify risk factors for subsequent mood changes (such as pre-existing depression) in order to exclude high risk patients from the surgery.[75]

As mentioned above, some PD patients suffer from personality changes and uncontrolled behaviours as a side effect of their drugs. These include problem gambling, reckless spending and increased sex drive. One of the big questions for the current evaluation of DBS is whether it can improve these symptoms as well. There is already some evidence that pathological behavioural addictions in PD can be reduced with DBS.[76, 77] For example, one patient who had led a successful professional life before being diagnosed with PD at the age of 44, started gambling with serious financial consequences after being started on dopaminergic medication and also developed hypersexuality. As a result of the DBS, his dose of dopaminergic medication could be reduced, and one year after surgery his hyperdopaminergic behaviours had disappeared and he commented:

> I was living like a mad man. I was irrational and unstable. I should have been locked up. But that's all over now – I'm free from all those vices. I have no more unhealthy thoughts, no more sick needs. Now I am at peace in all respects.[77]

For this patient, the DBS appears to have been a clear success story not only in relation to his motor symptoms but also in relation to his behaviour and mental stability. Others, however, fell into the opposite pattern when they were relieved of their hyperactivity and periods of elated mood (or hypomania). About one fifth of the patients in the most recent and largest study on this topic – a series of 63 French patients who received DBS in the STN – developed apathy, depression and anxiety, which are also sometimes reported amongst the side effects of DBS (or of the reduction of dopaminergic medication, which is a secondary aim of DBS from the neurological point of view). One central question in the evaluation is whether DBS has an overall beneficial effect on the patient's mental state and behaviour and just how disabling any change of behaviour is for the patient (and what effects it has on family and carers). When patients are in danger of gambling away their savings and engage in other reckless activities, such as dangerous driving or sexually inappropriate behaviour, this can have a serious impact on their health and well-being. However, other activities that are subsumed under the heading of behavioural addiction may be relatively innocuous compulsions or intended to compensate for some of the loss of function experienced by the patient in other domains. For example, in the French study the definition of behavioural addiction was rather broad and encompassed excessive engagement in the following activities during day or night: "philately, computer use, Internet surfing, gambling without money on the net or offline, bringing work home, housework, cooking, embroidery, decorating, do-it-yourself, gardening and taking work home."[77] All twelve patients who displayed these behaviours before the surgery were "cured" by the DBS treatment, but the question remains whether the risk of apathy and low mood is a price worth paying for this "normalisation" of behaviour. At the moment this is not a major question in the decision-making process before implanting DBS electrodes in PD patients because the main rationale for DBS is the better management of motor, rather than behavioural, problems. However, some researchers have advocated the use of subthalamic DBS for the treatment of Impulse Control Disorders unrelated to PD, and in this case the main target would be the behavioural symptoms. Although there is currently no evidence that DBS can actually improve impulse control in its own right (as opposed to indirectly by contributing to a dose reduction of dopaminergic medication in PD) some teams of neurosurgeons and neurologists or psychiatrists have started evaluating its use for several types of addiction, as will be discussed in Section 2.11. This brings back memories of a time in the, not so distant, past when surgical interventions were advocated for behaviour change across a wide range of domains.

2.9 Psychiatric surgery: from lobotomy to stereotactic control of behaviour

Lobotomy and leucotomy

If brain stimulation can have as profound an effect on behaviour as we have seen in Section 2.3, in both animals and humans, it would be entirely reasonable to ask whether abnormal behaviour can be treated by intervening directly at brain level. If a brain area or network is deemed to be hyper- or hypoactive in a mental or behavioural disorder, the most direct remedy might be through surgery. The surgical approach may not cure the underlying problem but may at least contain the dysfunctional activation and thus reduce symptoms. One example of this type of approach is callosotomy for severe intractable epilepsy. This procedure entails cutting the corpus callosum, the main connection between the two hemispheres of the brain. The aim is to contain the spread of epileptic activity to one hemisphere, which prevents the most severe forms of epileptic attacks. Callosotomies, which were common in the 1950s and 1960s, are now rarely, if ever, performed because epilepsy can be contained better by the drugs and other operations, such as cutting out the foci of epileptic activity directly, which have become available (see Section 2.1). Yet the effect on mental functions of such complete disconnection of the hemispheres was surprisingly subtle. There was certainly no indication that patients, in the main, developed dual personalities or became confused about who they were. Patients only showed deficits if they were challenged in experimental settings, where researchers could strictly control what type of stimuli a hemisphere could "see", and then showed patterns of behaviour that might be specifically associated with the left or right halves of the brain. For example most patients were unable to name objects presented in the left half of the visual field (and thus to the right hemisphere) because their language centre was in the disconnected left hemisphere. However, although they stated that they had not seen anything, they correctly reacted to these visual stimuli by pressing buttons with their left hand and thus were able to engage in the appropriate behaviour whenever they were entirely under the control of the same hemisphere. The fascinating history of split-brain research has been described in several books by one of its pioneers, Michael Gazzaniga. In his most recent book, *Who's in charge? Free will and the science of the brain*, he argues that split-brain experiments have shown that the right hemisphere is better at spatial and perceptual judgements than the left, but much less apt at integrative and associative processing of information and fails when a big picture is needed. Conversely, the left hemisphere, or more precisely what he calls the "interpreter module" within this hemisphere, tries to fit all available information into systems of cause and effect, which is generally a good way of trying to understand the world but can go wrong in cases where there is no cause and effect, just randomness. These considerations are of interest to anyone wanting to move from brain control to mind control because for the latter, ultimately, one would presumably have to target this interpreter module, which, according to Gazzaniga, provides us with the "personal narrative...that ties together all the disparate aspects of our conscious experience into a coherent whole".[78]

However, we do not need to worry that neuroscientists will, in the near future, be able to manipulate this module directly and through it our experience of being ourselves. No researcher has so far managed to localise this interpreter module or identify its network properties, and its manipulation by brain stimulation is therefore impossible at present. Incidentally, there are much more straightforward ways of hijacking the interpreter, as Gazzaniga convincingly points out, by manipulating the information it receives from the outside world, as has been done in numerous social psychology experiments.

Callosotomy was generally considered a clinical success for its time, despite being replaced by better drugs and more localised surgical procedures, and there were little if any concerns that it would control the mind. Conversely, another, now obsolete, procedure is lobotomy, which has a sinister reputation today. Attempts to control patients' brains – and minds – through surgery were widespread in psychiatry in the 1940s and 1950s, especially in the United States. Earlier attempts to treat mental illness by cutting out parts of the cortex or severing connections between cortical areas had been made by the Swiss psychiatrist Gottlieb Burckhardt in the 1880s and the Estonian surgeon Ludvig Puusepp in the early years of the 20th century. Burckhardt subscribed to the view, popular in the second half of the 19th century, that all mental illness had a primary organic basis and reasoned that, if abnormal behaviour arose from abnormal connections between sensory and motor fields in the cortex, taking out some of these connections should improve symptoms. However, he abandoned his programme after his reports on a small series of cases met with the disapproval of the international psychiatric community.[79]

The lobotomists of the 1930s–1950s initially received a much more positive public response. Lobotomy was the most famous psychosurgical intervention and its most famous proponent was Walter Jackson Freeman II (1895–1972).[44, 80, 81] Freeman was a neurologist frustrated by the lack of treatments available for his psychiatric patients – in those days many outpatients with mental health problems were seen by neurologists, whereas much of psychiatry was focused on work in the asylum. Freeman seized upon the opportunity to use a method developed by the Portuguese neurologist Egas Moniz (1874–1955), who shared the Nobel Prize in 1949 with Hess (see Section 1.3) "for his discovery of the therapeutic value of leucotomy in certain psychoses". From today's perspective it may have been more prudent to award him the Nobel Prize for his other main discovery, the cerebral angiogram (a way of depicting the brain's blood vessels on an X-ray), which is still in clinical use today.

Moniz's leucotomy was a relatively simple procedure that allowed the surgeon to cut the fibre tracts that connected the frontal lobes, the executive centres, with the rest of the brain. It was called leucotomy because essentially it cut off the white matter connections (Greek leukos=white) to the frontal lobe (Figure 2.8).

This procedure was originally intended for patients with severe melancholic depression or disabling obsessive thoughts and compulsive behaviours. However, it also became widely used in patients with schizophrenia, a psychiatric disease characterised by hearing voices, delusions, bizarre beliefs and actions and often a debilitating cognitive and social decline. One idea that emerged in the 1930s was that the most disturbing symptoms, including hallucinations and paranoia, were caused by a miswiring of the frontal lobe, and that cutting these connections might relieve the symptoms and allow the patients, who populated the large American asylums of the time, to be integrated into society. Several tens of thousands of psychiatric patients were operated on up until the 1950s in the USA, United Kingdom and many other countries. Freeman conducted the largest worldwide lobotomy programme, and his most famous patient was Rosemary Kennedy, the sister of the

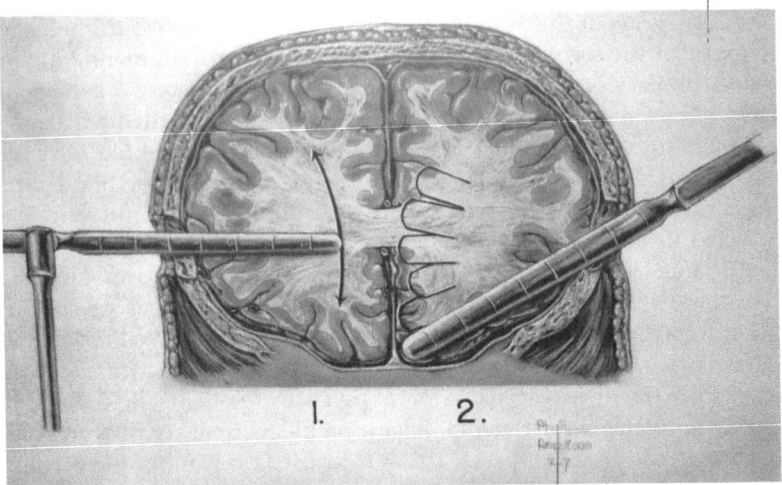

Figure 2.8   The standard leucotomy procedure in two steps (figure 15 from Freeman & Watts, 1950)[82]

future president John Fitzgerald Kennedy, although her outcome was not very good. He took the surgery directly into the asylums through his modifications of standard leucotomy, which enabled him to conduct the procedure through the orbit where the base of the skull is thin and can be pierced with an icepick-type instrument, saving the need to drill a hole in the skull (Figure 2.9). He practised several thousand of these transorbital lobotomies himself,[81] travelling from asylum to asylum. Freeman wrote:

> Transorbital lobotomy... abates the psychosis without producing any undesirable personality changes. Transorbital lobotomy is simple, quick, and safe. It is recommended particularly for psychiatrists in mental hospitals where major neurosurgical procedures are not available.[83]

Needless to say, the implication that interventions in the brain could be performed relatively easily by non-surgeons, psychiatrists even, angered many neurosurgeons of his (and later) times.

The initial reports on the outcomes of lobotomy stunned many psychiatrists. Patients who had been suffering from severe forms of paranoia and had to be detained in institutions for many years because of

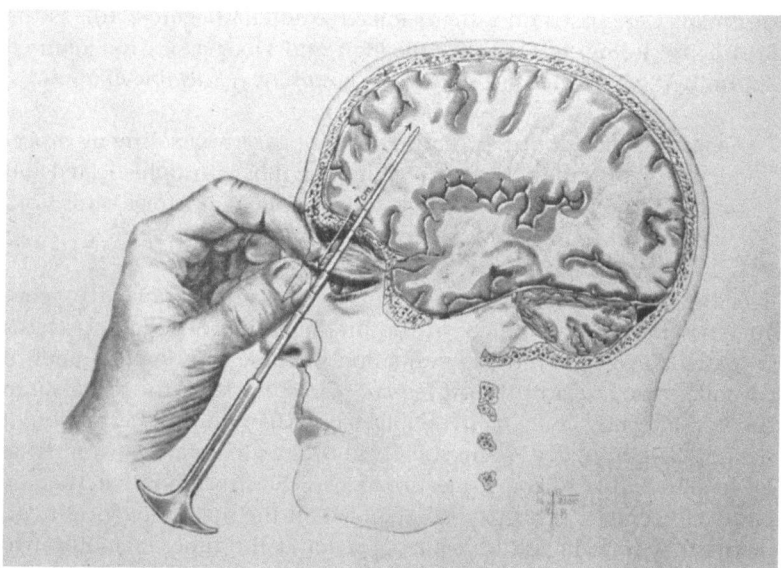

Figure 2.9 Depiction of transorbital leucotomy developed by Freeman (figure 20 from Freeman & Watts, 1950)[82]

violent tendencies became placid and outwardly undisturbed. However, they had to pay a high price because often the main reason for their more orderly behaviour was that the operation had reduced their drive and, in some cases, rendered them apathetic and oblivious to their environment. These personality changes also impacted upon the ability of patients to find employment, which was often cited as an important marker of the success of the procedure. As the American psychiatrists Lothar Kalinowsky and Paul Hoch pointed out in their 1961 textbook on *Somatic Treatments in Psychiatry*:

> Many of our patients who have shown rather poor results are employed in some family enterprise or by friends who, for various motives, are willing to put up with their shortcomings. They are often late for work or do not show up at all on days when they did not feel like working.[84]

The outcome of psychiatric surgery has been a matter of debate and controversy since its inception, and in many cases claims of successful treatment were based on rather subjective criteria (Figure 2.10), as the British psychologists Mark O'Callaghan and Douglas Carroll pointed out in their comprehensive survey *Psychosurgery: A Scientific Analysis*:

> Anecdotal testimonies of dramatic cure, bizarre assessment procedures (e.g. pre- and postoperative photographs), unsophisticated and casual methods of follow-up (e.g. the receipt of Christmas cards from a patient) and "amateur" statistics … are far from atypical.[85]

Even the Rorschach test, the projective personality test popular in psychoanalytic circles which relied on the interpretation of inkblot patterns by patients, was used in the evaluation of these early programmes of psychiatric surgery. In 1951 the *Journal of Mental Science*, the precursor to the *British Journal of Psychiatry*, published a paper on the "Evaluation of the Rorschach Test as a Prognostic Aid in the Treatment of Schizophrenia by Insulin Coma Therapy, Electronarcosis, Electroconvulsive Therapy and Leucotomy".[86] This paper assembled all the main biological treatments that were in use for schizophrenia at the time, including two treatments that operated through the induction of sleep by drastically

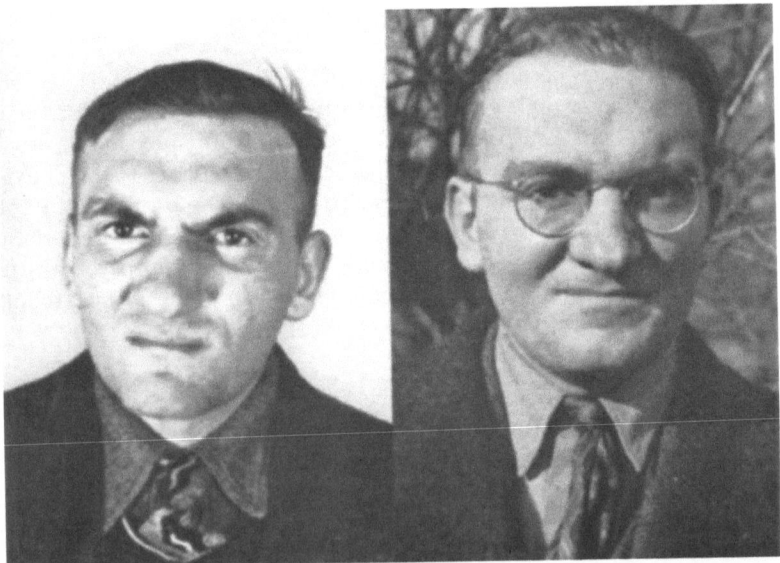

Figure 2.10   Example of pre- and postoperative photographs used as outcome measures to show the success of lobotomy (figure 58 from Freeman & Watts, 1950)[82]

lowering blood sugar (with administration of insulin) or by external high frequency electrical stimulation of the brain stem (electronarcosis). Insulin Coma Therapy and Electronarcosis were soon abandoned because of their medical risks and the availability of new antipsychotic drugs, and leucotomy suffered a similar fate. The only treatment on that list that still has a place in modern psychiatric treatment is Electroconvulsive Therapy (ECT).[87] It is important to note that the proponents of psychiatric surgery were by no means operating on the fringes of the psychiatry of their time. The leading professional psychiatric journals on both sides of the Atlantic, the *American* and *British Journals of Psychiatry*, for example, regularly carried articles on procedures for psychiatric surgery and reports on their outcome. The career of the author of the 1951 paper on the Rorschach test is a case in point. William Linford Llewelyn Rees, at the time a psychiatrist at the Whitchurch asylum in Cardiff, Wales, later had a distinguished academic career in London and became president of the British Royal College of Psychiatrists and the British Medical Association and Treasurer of the World Psychiatric Association.

Although we may now be inclined to view as rather amateurish some of the attempts of the 1940s and 1950s to evaluate the outcomes of psychiatric surgery and to identify the types of patients who would be most likely to benefit from it, it has to be acknowledged that lobotomy was one of the first treatments in psychiatry (and medicine in general) to be evaluated by formal follow-up studies. Some of these studies operated on a massive scale. The largest was a survey of leucotomies in England and Wales 1942–1954, conducted for the British Ministry of Health in 1961, which included over 10,000 patients. This survey was based on questionnaires sent to all hospitals where psychiatric surgery had been performed and asked for basic information about outcome, such as clinical gradings of patients who were still in hospital. However, as O'Callaghan and Carroll remarked, the "impression of patients' conditions before and after psychosurgery contained in case notes, being subjective in nature, hardly constitute a vigorous and objective evaluation of psychosurgery."[85]

Some prospective studies included a direct re-examination of the patients after several years, for example at the Maudsley Hospital in London or in the Columbia Greystone Project in New York. These more in-depth studies came to the conclusion that, overall, lobotomy had not produced any sizeable clinical benefits, but neither had it done major damage to cognitive functions and personality.[44] It has to be remembered, though, that it was an invasive procedure, accompanied by side effects of brain surgery, such as epilepsy, in up to 10% of cases.

Lobotomy fell out of favour in the mid-1950s and was soon superseded by the newly discovered antipsychotic drugs, which then ushered in the revolution in clinical psychiatry that Freeman had hoped to produce through lobotomy.

Behavioural surgery of the amygdala and hypothalamus

Although certainly the largest and most widely known, these leucotomy and lobotomy programmes were by no means the only effort to apply surgical methods in psychiatry. The newly developed stereotactic methods, which enabled less invasive but accurate approaches to deep brain structures, were used to selectively lesion areas that were deemed responsible for unwanted behaviours. Stereotactic lesions of the amygdala were used to control aggression and hyperactivity. Although these procedures now seem to have been abandoned (or replaced by DBS, as we will see in Section 2.11), over a thousand patients were treated with different forms of amygdalotomies until the late 1980s. For example, the Japanese neurosurgeon Dr Hirataro Narabayashi tried to treat irritability and other behavioural problems in the 1950s and 1960s by injecting oil into the amygdala on one or both sides of the brain.[88] He did not confine himself to any specific diagnostic group but operated on patients with epilepsy, children with developmental delay and patients who had retained brain damage from encephalitis (inflammation of the brain).[44] For example, he reported the case of a 12-year old boy who had suffered at the age of three from Japanese B encephalitis, a severe form of viral encephalitis with seizures and subsequent brain damage. He had lost his speech, which up to then had developed normally, and had great difficulty walking, with weakness on his right side. His behaviour before the operation was described as hyperirritable and excitable and he needed constant observation by his family. Brain imaging suggested that encephalitis had mainly affected his left hemisphere. This explained why speech and motor control of the right side, both functions commonly located in the left hemisphere, had been impaired. Narabayashi decided to destroy the amygdala on the right, the healthy side, guided by the rationale that "the activity of the healthy hemisphere was actually being modified by pathologic impulses originating from the atrophic, abnormal left hemisphere". The child was described as much calmer after the operation and able to "sit and play by himself" and no longer needed constant supervision.

Although some justification can perhaps be provided for such invasive behavioural interventions in patients with severe irreversible brain damage, other cases in Narabayashi's series clearly go beyond what would be deemed acceptable today (and should have raised concerns at the time). For example, he destroyed the left amygdala in a five-year old boy who had been diagnosed with "the hyperactive type of feeblemind-edness". This boy's – or his parents' – main problem was that he had an extremely short concentration span and had frequent temper tantrums. After the operation, "the hyperactivity had been abolished, and his entire attitude had become completely normal". Of the 60 patients whose operations Narabayashi reported, he classified 29 as "greatly improved, becoming calm, obedient and social adaptation being possible", and a further 22 as "moderately improved, easier to control, calm and with better concentration".[88] Along similar lines, Dr V Balasubramaniam, working at the General Hospital in Madras (now Chennai) destroyed both amygdalae of 115 patients with epilepsy or post-encephalitic brain damage for the purposes of calming them down, a procedure he termed "sedative neurosurgery".[44]

The other main target of neurosurgery for behaviour disorders was the hypothalamus. Another Japanese neurosurgeon, Keiji Sano (1920–2011) promoted the use of lesions in the posterior medial hypothalamus to control aggressive behaviour. He was explicitly guided by Hess's distinc-tion of trophotropic and ergotropic zones in the hypothalamus. Sano thought that aggression and rage were produced by an imbalance between these hypothalamic systems (in favour of the ergotropic) and that lesioning the ergotropic zones ought to restore this balance and control aggression. He localised his target area by electrical stim-ulation and placed the lesion in the area where he evoked the most marked sympathetic response (a rise in blood pressure and heart rate and a widening of the pupils). At the Second International Symposium on Stereoencephalotomy (=stereotactic brain surgery) held in Vienna in 1965 Sano reported on 22 patients where he had conducted this procedure bilaterally (except in one case with atrophy of one hemi-sphere where only the non-atrophied side was operated on). They all suffered from epilepsy and intractable violent behaviour. His youngest patient was four. He reported "satisfactory calming effects" in all cases. Specifically, he described changes in emotion and personality: "The patient became markedly calm, passive and tractable, showing decreased spontaneity."[89]

Even those cases with the most successful outcomes, the amygdaloto-mies and hypothalamotomies in patients whose behavioural problems were mostly caused by severe brain damage and accompanied by learning difficulties or cognitive impairment, were hardly magical cures. It may be useful to consider the two patients reported in a paper from the 1990s who were followed up with modern techniques.[90] Both patients were operated on as young men. One patient had developed normally until the age of ten, when he suffered encephalitis caused by the herpes simplex virus. He subsequently suffered from complex partial seizures and impulsive and aggressive behaviour. Although his seizures could be controlled well enough with anti-epileptic drugs, the rage attacks continued and made it impossible for him to go on with his schooling. He had to live in an institution from the age of 13. He had a bilateral amygdalotomy when he was 19. After the operation his assaultive outbursts went down from seven per month to about one every other month. However, when they did occur, they were rather dramatic, including "self-abuse (e.g. stabbing neck with pencil, slamming head against wall, drinking liquid laundry detergent), destruction of property (e.g. breaking windows, tearing clothing off himself, throwing and breaking ceramics, destroying furniture), and assaults (e.g. biting, kicking, hitting, and stabbing others, resulting in broken bones, teeth, dentures, and glasses)". Ten years after the operation and 16 years after his initial hospitalisation he could finally be transferred from hospital to a care home.

The outcome of the other patient was even more limited. This patient had suffered a chickenpox encephalitis aged eight months and subsequently developed complex partial seizures, which were well controlled with medication. However, in his teenage years he also developed rage attacks, which made it necessary for him to live in an institution from age 13. Because his aggressive outbursts did not respond to any drug treatment he received a bilateral amygdalotomy when he was 21. Although his "temper tantrums" diminished in frequency, they could still be severe when they did happen: "In late 1996, D.B.B. assaulted the supervisor of his personal care home, causing the supervisor to suffer significant head injury (coma lasting several days), multiple broken bones, and loss of an eye. Bystanders reported that D.B.B. stopped this assault only after being restrained by other residents of the personal care home." Furthermore, his non-aggressive impulsive behaviour ("running away, spending all his money immediately after receiving it, compulsive alcohol consumption") increased after the operation. In his case, the psychiatric surgery was considered to have failed.

Operations on sexual offenders

Now let us turn to the following scenario: how about a person suffering from urges to engage in indecent or even criminal acts consenting to a surgical procedure that relieves him from these urges and allows him to comply with social and legal norms? The classic example would be that of an abusive paedophile who has spent time in jail for child abuse and now, after his release, would like to support his rehabilitation with an operation that removes his abnormal sexual interests. In the 1960s and 1970s German neurosurgeons developed an operation that was intended to relieve abnormal sexual urges. They targeted the hypothalamus, which, as we discussed in Section 1.3, is the main central control area of the hormonal system. They inferred from animal experiments that some aspects of the hypersexuality displayed by monkeys after amygdala lesions resembled the deviant sexual behaviour of humans. On the basis of evidence that another lesion, this time placed in the ventromedial nucleus of the hypothalamus, normalised the animal's sexual drive, they explored a similar approach in humans. The approach of the German surgeons was to insert an electrode through a stereotactic apparatus into the hypothalamus. The target area could be localised in patients who were awake because it is very close to the main visual pathway, the optic tract, and electrical stimulation thus induces the perception of flashes of light. The surgeons then moved the electrode into its target position and applied a stronger electrical current which was intended to destroy the "sex-behaviour-centre", believed to be located in this area, the ventro-medial nucleus (see Figure 2.3).

The available reports[91] from the four German centres where this operation was conducted document the case histories of about 75 patients. The majority of patients were homosexual paedophiles who had been convicted of sexual offences. It is well known, and still a matter of considerable public debate today, that paedophiles who have offended have a high risk of reoffending and are often tormented by their sexual drive. Although their sexual preferences are difficult to change, their drive can often be controlled reasonably well with drugs that counteract the male sex hormone testosterone the, so-called, anti-androgens. However, the patients of the German surgeons had either not responded to such chemical castration or had found the side effects intolerable. One remaining option to reduce their libido and possibly cure them from their abnormal urges was surgical castration. According to German law this required both the patient's consent and the approval of a medical board. Although this approval had been given for several of these patients they still opted for the brain surgery. One consideration might have been that, if they could obtain the required change in sexual preferences and behaviour but keep their masculinity, the brain surgery would actually be the less invasive option.

The first patient of the neurologist Fritz Douglas Roeder in Goettingen, a 52-year old unmarried businessman who led a withdrawn and outwardly unremarkable life, was operated on in 1962. He had first been convicted of sexual abuse of minors in 1950. He was jailed for one and a half years but committed further sexual abuse after his release, which led to further jail sentences. On one occasion he even abused three children while he was on the way to his lawyer. The risk he posed to the public was deemed sufficiently high to warrant detention in a psychiatric hospital after the end of his sentence. His psychiatrists uncovered important details of his past, for example that he had suffered abuse himself at the hand of a teacher when he was 13, but they felt that a lengthy psychotherapy would be unlikely to produce much benefit. This was the point when surgical destruction of the presumed sex centre in the brain was considered. The patient hoped that this would make him indifferent to the attraction of the male body. He also expressed the hope that a successful surgical intervention would spare him detention in a psychiatric hospital. After his operation, a destruction of the ventromedial nucleus of the hypothalamus on the right side of the brain, he recovered well, without major cognitive deficits or hormonal changes. The most important change was that his sexual interest in children had disappeared. He moved to another city, started relationships with women, pursued a successful business career and committed no further crimes until his death in 1974 from tuberculosis. Although in this, and the majority of other cases, criminal prosecution and a wish to avoid further detention were certainly strong motivating factors for agreeing to the procedure, other patients sought a surgeon's help even in the absence of any such incentives.

The functional neurosurgery group at Hamburg University, followed up all their 28 hypothalamotomy patients over the course of 12 years.[92] Nine of these patients, of whom all but one were males, had a history of paedophilia, others had suffered from other paraphilias (exhibitionism, fetishism) or had committed rape on women or girls. All but three of them had been convicted of mostly sexual offences. Most patients underwent hypothalamotomy on the non-dominant side of the brain only. If the initial procedure was ineffective, some patients had a second operation on the dominant side and two decided to undergo surgical castration; 24 out of the 28 patients experienced a considerable and lasting reduction of sexual drive, and 23 reported a clear reduction in the stimulating effect of sexual cues. The authors interpreted this as a vindication of their clinical approach, which had specifically targeted patients who were experiencing abnormal arousal from such cues.

Although 20 patients had no further convictions, five did have further convictions for sexual offences (including one homicide, the patient described in more detail below) and three had new convictions for non-sexual offences, such as theft. Although some patients developed lasting heterosexual relationships after the operation, maintaining a stable relationship remained a major difficulty for many of them. The development of their work situation was more positive, with most managing to get more stable jobs. Eight patients moved into more responsible and qualified positions, and 24 developed interests in hobbies, whereas they had previously largely been occupied with their sexual obsessions.

As indicated by the follow-up study from Hamburg, the hypothalamotomy did not provide absolute protection against sexual reoffending. This became clear most dramatically in the case of Bernd Lichtenberg, reported in the German weekly *Der Spiegel* on 28 April 1980. Lichtenberg, who was operated on in Hamburg in 1976, had a history of abusing boys who were around the age of 10. If they resisted he would threaten to kill them. He had already been convicted for sexual crimes when he was 17, but all therapeutic efforts were in vain. The operation seemed initially to reduce his obsessive thoughts about young boys, and Lichtenberg even got engaged to a woman when he was released on probation. Up to this point his sexual drive had been curbed by chemical castration, but he was now eager to stop taking the anti-androgen, although this treatment was one of his probation conditions. When he stopped this libido-reducing treatment the authorities were slow to intervene and he ended up killing a 10-year old boy whom he had approached sexually. This demonstration of the fallibility of the surgical "cure" for paedophilia was used by parts of the German media to discredit the procedure, although its use had already effectively ceased by the end of 1976.

Operating on the brain to change someone's sexual orientation, even with the sole intent of relieving a person's own suffering and with their full consent, had immediately raised ethical and legal concerns in Germany and internationally. Valenstein, in his 1973 book, commented:

> There is little in the description of the cases operated on by Roeder and his colleagues, or the underlying animal research, that can even begin to justify the extreme confidence they express in their psycho-surgical procedure. ... Clearly, this is an example of a group adopting a psychosurgical procedure based on an arbitrary selection from the total animal data available and then reporting their clinical results in a completely inadequate form. No indication has been presented

that these investigators have or intend to employ the type of behavior testing necessary for an objective evaluation of postoperative changes.

This wholesale dismissal of the German programme is interesting because Valenstein was much less critical of Narabayashi's or Balasubramaniam's surgical programmes for behaviour control. Valenstein's main argument against Roeder and his colleagues was:

> When allowance is made for the fact that the patients generally want to change their behavior, there is no reason to believe that the surgery produced a change in sexual orientation. The major effect of the surgery seems to be a general reduction of sexual drive to the point where it is possible for the patient to control his deviant behavior.[44]

From today's point of view, however, Valenstein's critique might actually be seen as a support for the procedure. Later follow-up studies did endorse the view that the main effect of hypothalamotomy was to curb the sexual drive rather than change the sexual orientation.[93] Whilst we would probably be more reluctant to endorse an operation that completely changes a person's sexual preferences (and thus an integral part of their personality) we might accept interventions that enable people to deal with their preferences in a socially acceptable manner.

Although an expert committee of the German Federal Health Agency published recommendations for the safeguarding of patient interests and for a scientific evaluation of neurosurgery for sexual disorders in 1978, no further operations were conducted because the public debate had become too toxic and clinicians were reluctant to be linked to psychiatric surgery programmes. Interestingly, stereotactic neurosurgery for sexual disorders remains legal in Germany, provided a patient has the capacity to consent and is not coerced, and would probably be legal in most other jurisdictions provided these safeguards are in place. Yet, although sexual offenders still pose a major problem to legal systems because of the high rate of reoffending, and although treatment is very difficult and success rates are low, there has been virtually no consideration of a revival of the surgical method. This is interesting from a political and societal point of view because other very restrictive measures, notably preventive detention, are being considered in several countries instead. We will revisit this issue in the wider context of the political and social debate on surgical control of behaviour in Chapter 4.

2.10 Psychiatric surgery today

Surgical approaches to OCD and depression

Although full-scale lobotomy was abandoned in the 1950s, other ways of cutting connections between parts of the brain for the treatment of mental disorders lived on and some are still in use today. In 1949 the French neurosurgeon Jean Talairach presented the stereotactic anterior capsulotomy (Figure 2.11), which was popularised by the Swedish neurosurgeon Lars Leksell, who used it on over 100 patients in the 1950s. A large portion of the fibres connecting the limbic system with the frontal lobe travel through the basal ganglia region of the brain, and in this bottleneck they form a joint tract in the anterior limb of the internal capsule. Procedures to cut this tract, for example by applying heat and thus destroying the tissue (thermal surgery), are called anterior capsulotomy. This procedure also destroys a part of the medial forebrain bundle, which carries connections between dopaminergic midbrain areas and the frontal lobe. Because the connections between the frontal lobe and the limbic system are deemed particularly important for emotion and anxiety regulation, this procedure has mostly been tried in depression and obsessive compulsive disorder (OCD) with reasonable clinical improvement rates.[94] Recently, non-invasive radiosurgery with gamma rays (gamma knife) has also been used for applications in OCD, but problems with intracerebral bleeds have halted this programme.

Another approach, initially suggested by MacLean's teacher John Fulton in the 1940s as a less invasive alternative to lobotomy, targeted the fibres between the limbic system and frontal lobes in the cingulum (cingulotomy) (Figure 2.11).

The cingulotomy procedure was initially mainly used in chronic pain patients who did not respond to other treatments. The rationale was that the cingulate cortex, which is connected to the rest of the brain via the cingulum bundle, is centrally involved in the processing of pain, and seems to be particularly important for its affective component, the aversive experience associated with pain. However, it turned out that cingulotomy was most effective for pain patients who were also suffering from depression or anxiety. The next step was to evaluate bilateral cingulotomy for OCD and other mental disorders. This was done in a large study over several decades at the Massachusetts General Hospital in Boston, USA, in almost 200 patients. This study was reported by Harvard University neurosurgeon H. Thomas Ballantine in 1987, who found over half the patients to be improved after surgery.[95] However, these evaluations were still conducted in an era in which the outcome of psychiatric patients was judged by clinical impression, rather than

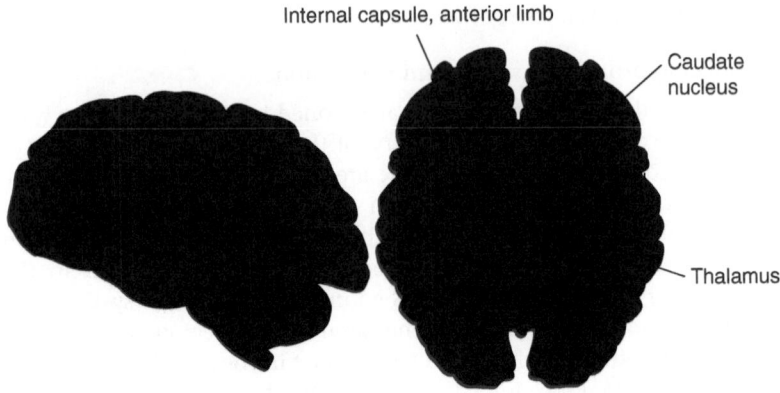

Internal capsule, anterior limb

Caudate nucleus

Thalamus

Figure 2.11   Main targets of psychiatric surgery today

Note: Anterior capsulotomy (1), cingulotomy (2) and subcaudate tractotomy (3) shown on schematic drawings. Subcaudate tractotomy targets tracts from the orbitofrontal cortex to subcortical areas that travel through the zone between the caudate nucleus and the amygdala. The combination of cingulotomy and subcaudate tractotomy is called limbic leucotomy.

formal rating scales (which is not necessarily bad, but rating scales are somewhat less prone to the bias of the treating clinician). Over the next 20 years, the Harvard neurosurgeons evaluated their cingulotomy programme for OCD more formally. The surgeons produced bilateral lesions of around 3 cm in length in the anterior part of the cingulate gyrus with the intention of severing the fibre tracts travelling through the cingulum bundle. If the patients did not improve they added a lesion in the subgenual cingulate, thus converting the procedure to the, so-called, limbic leucotomy (Figure 2.11). About half of the 64 patients operated on had responded after five years. Treatment response was defined as an improvement of at least 35% on the standard assessment scale for OCD, the Yale Brown Obsessive Compulsive Scale (YBOCS). However, two patients in this group committed suicide. Suicidal ideation, which can occur as part of a severe OCD, was reported as already present before surgery.[96] Suicide as a potential side effect of treatment for mental disorders, which carry a suicide risk in themselves, is notoriously difficult to evaluate. For example, a very active debate concerns the question of whether suicides observed in trials of antidepressant drugs are effects of the treatment or of the disorder. At the very least, new patients need to be made aware of the occurrence of suicide in previous trials of DBS and psychiatric surgery.

The efficacy of surgical intervention seems to be similar in OCD and depression, where about half the patients showed clinical improvement after the surgery in a recent series of anterior capsulotomy cases.[97] A slightly higher response rate was reported in a cohort of patients from Australia with treatment-resistant depression, who had undergone a bilateral orbitomedial leucotomy, a stereotactic procedure where fibres from the limbic system to the anterior portion of the frontal lobe are cut when they travel through the area of the frontal lobe above the orbit. There was a clinical improvement in 16 of the 23 patients operated on between 1973 and 1995, on whom detailed clinical data were available, with five even recovering fully.[98] Interestingly, clinical improvement was apparent within days or weeks of surgery, although full recovery took several months (and sometimes required a second operation). However, six out of the original 76 patients in this case series had committed suicide, reinforcing the need to monitor this potential side effect of surgical interventions in psychiatry.

Some patients report that surgical intervention for depression or OCD has effectively changed their lives. Patients who before the intervention had to spend much of their time in psychiatric hospitals, undergoing intensive treatment with antidepressant drugs and electroconvulsive therapy, could return to their homes and manage with much lower doses of drugs (although rarely completely without). These patients generally feel that being freed of the gloom of depression is worth the side effects, which can include fatigue and weight gain. Increased appetite and weight gain are amongst the most commonly reported side effects of both the newer stereotactic approaches and the classic leucotomies, where up to 90% of patients experienced an often dramatic weight gain.[99]

Surprisingly, cutting off the connections to the frontal lobe and limbic system through these procedures seems to have relatively few consequences for cognitive functions. However, cognitive side effects may have been under-reported because standard tests of intelligence and cognitive performance were not sensitive enough to the specific deficits in planning and action control that can be produced by frontal lobe lesions, and a considerable number of patients did complain about memory problems. The surgery is relatively safe in other respects, although small localised cerebral bleeds are relatively common and post-operative epilepsy occurred in about 10% of patients after the earlier, more invasive operations. This has come down considerably with stereotactic interventions. In nearly a thousand cingulotomies performed at the Massachusetts General Hospital in Boston, the seizure rate was only 1% and no patient died from surgical complications.[100]

One central question is why patients might benefit from psychiatric surgery. One possibility is that such a radical procedure also has a strong placebo effect. The placebo effect is based on the patient's expectation that a drug or other intervention will work. It can be very powerful, for example in the treatment of pain or indeed in that of depression. It has even been estimated that 80% of the effects of antidepressant drugs are attributable to the placebo effect (which does not mean that one can just replace the drug because the placebo effect is much weaker if people are told that they are receiving a placebo). Thus, some of the benefits of psychosurgery could be attributable to a placebo effect. After all, a brain operation is no mean feat, and if I have a structure removed on both sides of my brain I really want this operation to work out. Whether a treatment works better than a placebo is normally tested by comparing the treatment in question, say a drug, with another one that smells and tastes the same but does not have the active chemical ingredients, the placebo. In psychiatric surgery this information is generally not available because trials with "fake" surgery have rarely been conducted (and, admittedly, are not as straightforward as drug trials with a placebo control).

One exception is the series of anterior cingulate lesions conducted by neurosurgeon Dr Kenneth Livingston on psychiatric patients at the Veterans Administration Hospital at Roseburg, Oregon between 1949 and 1953.[44] Several of his, approximately, 100 cases received sham operations, either because they did not cooperate during the surgery, which was conducted under local anaesthesia only, or because it had been planned in this way in advance. Neither patients nor staff knew who had received a sham operation (and the patients were certainly not aware that they were, in effect, part of a single-blind controlled trial, which is a major ethical problem with this study). The reported outcomes were much better for the patients with the real cingulotomy than for those who received the sham operation, and the latter group indeed received the real operation in a further session a few months later. Although this was not a placebo-controlled trial according to today's standards, it provided some evidence for the specific effects of focal lesions. Still, the placebo effect may play an important role in the, often stunning, improvements in depression or OCD after surgery, but we also have to remember that these patients were only included in the surgery programme because they were otherwise treatment-refractory. That is, they had not responded to the (real or placebo) effects of the standard treatments available.

Is having a brain operation that only improves symptoms in 50% of cases, through largely unknown mechanisms, and possibly not better than a placebo intervention, a price worth paying? Only the patients themselves can tell. They may not care that we do not know why psychosurgery works (we actually know equally little about the reasons why antidepressant drugs work) and may see a 50% chance of recovering from a lifelong disabling illness, which has not been improved by several courses of treatment with drugs that can have side effects that are more severe than those of surgery. Destructive surgery of this type for mental disorders will certainly always only be a treatment of last resort, only to be considered if all other viable treatment options have been exhausted. In addition, it will generally require approval by an ethics committee or similar official body. For example in the UK, the Mental Health Act (section 57) specifies that the performance of psychiatric surgery requires, in addition to the patient's consent, that a panel appointed by the Home Secretary certifies the patient's capacity to provide consent and that the responsible clinician consults with two other professionals, one of whom must be a nurse, regarding the suitability of the treatment.

Surgery for addiction – a controversial path

Whereas psychiatric surgery in the USA and the UK is presently only performed in patients with depression and OCD, other countries have a wider range of indications. Although addiction was not a main target of the original leucotomy procedures, several groups performed surgery on patients with alcohol and opiate addiction in the 1960s and 1970s. The German proponents of hypothalamotomy, for example, also operated on patients with alcohol dependence and reported some encouraging initial results, although they also observed a number of relapses. A larger programme of cingulotomies for addiction was started by Balasubramaniam in India. Interestingly, cingulotomies were still offered to patients with alcohol or heroin addiction in Russia in the late 1990s and early 2000s. The surgical technique was slightly different from the standard approach because the surgeons at the Institute of the Human Brain in St Petersburg used cooling probes, rather than the heat produced by electrocoagulation, to destroy the fibre tract but the neuroanatomical effects were similar to those of the cingulotomies performed by Balasubramaniam or by Ballantine in his OCD programme. The therapy offered by the St Petersburg neurosurgeons was greeted initially with enthusiasm in the international press. On 7 February 1999 the *Observer*,

a leading British Sunday paper, carried a piece by Tom Whitehouse entitled "Russian addicts cured by surgery. Removing part of the brain under
local anaesthetic is a revolutionary cure that seems to work." It reported
on the case of a 19-year old heroin addict who had been cured – at least
for the time being – of her drug habit and was planning to return to
University. And it cited the head of the programme, Sviatoslav Medvedev,
as saying: "Addiction is a kind of obsession . ....There's a kind of circle in
the brain which has to be cut. That's our task."

However, just over three years later the picture changed after a patient
complained of side effects and the programme was halted. Nick Paton
Walsh wrote in *The Guardian*, the sister newspaper of the *Observer*, on
9 August 2002 under the heading "Russia bans brain surgery on drug
addicts":

> A series of controversial brain operations pioneered by St Petersburg
> scientists as a cure to drug addiction has been halted by Russian
> authorities after a patient complained of damaging side-effects...The
> patient claimed he had suffered headaches as a result of the operation,
> which also failed to cure him of his addiction. The court awarded him
> the cost of the surgery, about £5,000. Russian authorities then halted
> use of the procedure on the grounds that it was experimental and had
> not been licensed by the health ministry.

However, the surgeons themselves claimed good results.[101] Of the 187
patients with heroin addiction operated on, whom they could follow-up
over two years (just over half of their overall patient sample), 43%
reported full abstinence. Although this means that 57% of the patients
relapsed this would still be a relatively good two-year outcome compared
to conventional (psychological and medical) interventions for addiction, although at the cost of an invasive procedure. However, we have to
bear in mind that the published abstinence rate was based on the self-
reports of patients (who may have many reasons for under-reporting
their heroin use) rather than laboratory tests.

Moreover, cingulotomy, quite apart from the ethical and safety considerations, is perhaps not the ideal neurobiological approach to addiction. Medvedev's assumption that "addiction is a kind of obsession" is
certainly not shared by all researchers. Commenting in the specialist
journal *Lancet Neurology* in 2002, Harvard psychiatrist Edwin Cassem
expressed the general view that, "We do not classify addictions with
obsessive-compulsive disorders." However, he did not categorically
exclude the possibility that an intervention affecting the same tracts

would have therapeutic benefits in both OCD and addiction: "Any limbic circuit finds its way to the septum and accumbens."[102]

It is certainly true that one needs to beware of simplistic analogies between OCD and substance addiction. Addiction has three key components: the joyful experience of the consumption, or liking; the urge to obtain the drug, or wanting, sometimes also expressed as craving; and the habitual, almost compulsive use, which can perhaps be best observed in inveterate smokers. Only the last aspect bears close resemblance to OCD symptoms, whereas liking and wanting are probably subserved by other brain circuits. At least this is suggested by animal experiments, which provide evidence for a liking circuit, consisting of hedonic hotspots (and related to the opioid group of neurotransmitters),[103] and a wanting circuit, incorporating the dopaminergic motivational system. These two circuits indeed overlap at the level of the nucleus accumbens, which has also been the main target for DBS in addiction, both in the few human[104] and in the much larger number of animal studies. Surgical destruction of the nucleus accumbens has been used by at least two groups in China to treat opiate addiction.[105] One study from Xi'an followed up 60 patients who had undergone bilateral ablation of the nucleus accumbens. Almost 50% had remained abstinent after five years. In this case, the reports of abstinence were confirmed by urine testing for morphine. Although such low relapse rates are impressive compared with other treatments for opiate addiction, the functional outcome did not keep pace. The abstinent group only showed a marginal improvement in depression scores, and although slightly more people in both groups were in paid employment after five years than before the surgery, this effect was the same for the patients who remained abstinent and for those who relapsed.[106] Because the nucleus accumbens is a central part of the motivation and reward pathways, one would expect a lesion in this area to lead to apathy, fatigue and loss of interest, which was indeed observed in a considerable number of patients. Some also lost their interest in sexual activities. Almost half of the patients developed a milder temperament, which evokes some of the descriptions of postoperative placidity in the earlier lobotomy literature.

2.11 Will DBS replace psychiatric surgery?

OCD and Tourette's syndrome

A main conceptual advantage of DBS over surgery is that the stimulation parameters can be adjusted to the clinical needs of the individual patient, and even dynamically adapted to clinical states. In psychiatry, DBS is principally performed in OCD, which can be a very disabling condition. For example, some patients just cannot leave the house because they have to go back to check that all electrical appliances are turned off or wash their hands over and over again. Many patients also suffer from highly distressing obsessive thoughts and ruminations and worry constantly that they may do major damage to themselves or others. In many patients the course of the disease is chronic and symptoms do not respond well to medication.

DBS of various parts of the basal ganglia, for example the nucleus accumbens, subthalamic nucleus or the ventral capsule, has improved OCD symptoms in some patients.[94] However the medical world requires formal trials in order to accept a new treatment as effective. Because of the possibility of a placebo effect such trials always have to include control conditions. There are ethical problems in just inserting electrodes without using them, but one option is to compare the symptoms and general well-being of patients while the electrodes are switched on and while they are switched off (which the patients would not normally notice because there are no sensory receptors in the brain). Because people could simply get addicted to brain stimulation (see Section 2.3) it is important not just to start by stimulating for several months and then switching off for several months but also to proceed in the reverse order. The results of one such cross-over trial, with 16 OCD patients who had electrodes implanted into the subthalamic nucleus bilaterally, was published in 2008 in the *New England Journal of Medicine*, the most widely read medical journal in the world.[107] The symptom scores during the stimulation phases were significantly lower than during the off phases, but still amounted to OCD of moderate severity. Furthermore, several patients experienced surgical complications and some developed manic symptoms before the stimulation parameters were finally adjusted. This formal trial thus paints a slightly more sobering picture than the seen in some of the first patients. Furthermore, even in this design, all patients initially undergo a two-month stimulation period where the final electrical parameters are adjusted for each individual. Thus we cannot completely rule out that patients become addicted in some way to the electrical stimulation during this parameter-setting period and develop withdrawal symptoms during the ensuing off phase.

Tourette's syndrome (GTS), first formally described by the French neurologist Gilles de la Tourette in 1885, is another disabling condition that may improve after DBS. GTS is characterised by a combination of compulsive behaviour, such as the urge to utter obscenities (*koprolalia*), and uncontrolled movements of the head or limbs, so-called motor tics.

It often starts in childhood or adolescence, and about half of the patients are symptom-free by the time they reach adulthood. However, those whose symptoms persist often suffer from major psychiatric comorbidities such as OCD or ADHD, and can also develop physical injuries as a consequence of their forceful involuntary head or neck movements, such as retinal detachment or injuries to their spinal cord.[108] Needless to say, the utterance of obscenities and urges to repeat the words uttered by other people or themselves (*echolalia*) causes embarrassment and severely impairs their capacity for social interaction and normal careers.

The cause of GTS is unknown. Because of the prominence of motor symptoms it is commonly classified as a neurological disorder, but psychiatric problems may be even more important for the resulting social disability. Dysfunction of the basal ganglia has been implicated in GTS, and DBS of targets in the basal ganglia – the internal pallidum, nucleus accumbens or thalamus – indeed leads to some reduction of both the motor tics and *koprolalia*. Because the main established treatment with antipsychotic drugs is not very effective there may be scope for an increased use of DBS in this patient group. However, as in PD, some patients developed psychological side effects. such as hypomania, impaired impulse control or suicidal tendencies.

Depression

In 2005, the first study of DBS in depression was published in which a group from Toronto, Canada, implanted electrodes below the subgenual part of the cingulate cortex, where it is nested below the knee (Latin: *genu*) of the corpus callosum. They selected six patients with a long history of depression (between five and thirty years duration) who had not responded to a variety of treatments, including combinations of antidepressant drugs and ECT. The surgeons inserted the electrodes into both hemispheres and the stimulation parameters were similar to those in Parkinson's disease, with the aim of attenuating the presumed overactivity of the targeted area. All patients experienced changes in their mental state immediately after stimulation started, which is interesting because they cannot have felt it in any ordinary way as the brain is devoid of pain or other sensory receptors. They reported a general calming effect, heightened awareness and a sharpening of visual perception. The study was also considered to be a (preliminary) success in clinical terms because four out of the six patients responded to the intervention after the six month trial. A treatment response was defined as an improvement of 50% on a standard clinical scale, which is a criterion often used in antidepressant drug trials.

Since this first report from 2005 several slightly larger studies have investigated the effect of DBS in depression, although the overall number reported worldwide is probably still only around 100 patients.[109] The studies used different stimulation sites: the subgenual cingulate as in the first report; or two subcortical regions (nucleus accumbens or ventral internal capsule) familiar from DBS work in OCD. The number of responders did not depend substantially on the stimulated area and was generally between 30% and 50%.[110–112] The largest study so far is an ongoing crossover trial with 200 patients, half of whom will start with six months off stimulation before going on to receive the active stimulation.[113]

The most recent addition to the target areas of DBS for depression has been the MFB, based on the classic animal experiments by Olds discussed above. A German team working with neurosurgeon Volker Coenen recently reported the results from their first seven patients with treatment-refractory depression, in whom they implanted electrodes bilaterally into the MFB just after its exit from the ventral tegmental area in the midbrain.[114] They stimulated the MFB with relatively low intensity and observed a remarkable reduction in depressive symptoms after just one week, which is a short period for antidepressant effects since antidepressant drugs normally take several weeks to work. Contrary to other interventions which produce immediate antidepressant effects – ECT, sleep deprivation or single doses of the drug ketamine – their effects were sustained over several weeks, and even after several months four patients were classified as having remitted from their depression. As is the case with all DBS studies, there is a possibility that these improvements were largely due to a placebo effect. After all, DBS is an invasive procedure and patients' expectations of the surgery are high. Furthermore, depression is a relapsing-remitting illness, and thus some spontaneous improvement over time would normally be expected. However, the German team also described plausible instant effects of the MFB stimulation, which they observed when they were localising the target site during the operation. All patients showed, what they described as, increased appetitive motivation. The patients tried to change their head position and make eye contact with the psychologist who was testing them, and also became more vigilant. However they did not report an immediate pleasurable experience, which was in keeping with the experience of Heath, as discussed in Section 2.3, who failed to induce hedonic responses in the more anterior parts of the MFB in humans. The German team applied an interesting distinction between wanting and liking to their findings, which is often used in motivation research. The MFB stimulation induced a non-specific wanting but no explicit liking of its effects, which is potentially important when considering the addictive potential of such treatments.

Although DBS is starting to become an established treatment for very severe and otherwise treatment-refractory OCD, it does have side effects and will only provide partial relief for most patients. Its use in depression is still in an early state of clinical development, and further controlled studies are needed to determine whether it will become an accepted treatment option for otherwise treatment-refractory depression. Although response rates thus far have been good, there were also surgical complications (although they were classified as not being serious) and at least one suicide (although the study team maintained that it was unrelated to the intervention). Psychiatric surgery has so far not been replaced by DBS and the annual intervention numbers for both groups of procedures are very low compared to the huge number of patients across the globe suffering from some form of depression (estimated to be several hundred million). At the time of writing just under 300 psychiatric patients had been included in published DBS studies worldwide.[115]

Recently some research groups have also considered the use of DBS for the treatment of addiction, although very few patients have so far actually been stimulated.[104] For example, two patients with opiate addiction who underwent DBS of the nucleus accumbens in Cologne, Germany, continued to abstain from heroin and methadone during two years of stimulation (but continued consumption of other drugs).[116] The scientific basis for this procedure is largely derived from animal studies. Animals can be made addicted to a substance by giving them unlimited access to, for instance, cocaine. Their level of addiction can then be tested by their behaviour in contexts where the substance is available. For example, in a conditioned place preference experiment they will spend considerably more time in a part of the cage where they can drink the substance in question than in a part where only a control drink, for example sucrose, is available. This drug seeking behaviour can be abolished in experimental animals with DBS of the nucleus accumbens.[117] On this basis, and spurred on by encouraging reports from some of the case studies where addictive behaviour improved after DBS, some authors recommended starting trials of DBS in addiction in selected groups of patients. However, bioethicists have argued that this would be premature, and that more evidence from animal studies about suitable anatomical targets would be needed first.[118]

The group of neurosurgeons that developed DBS of the subgenual cingulate for depression have recently also applied this technique in patients with anorexia nervosa, whose low weight had not improved under several standard therapies. They implanted electrodes below the subgenual cingulate gyrus on both sides of the brain in six female patients. Treatment success (weight gain) was measured by changes on the body mass index (BMI). The BMI is calculated by dividing one's weight (in kilograms) by the height squared (in square metres). Thus, a person with a height of 1.50 cm (approximately 5 ft) and a weight of 33.7 kg (approximately 5 st) would have a BMI of approximately 15. The normal range is between 18.5 and 25, and all six patients started from pre-operative values below 18.5. After DBS, two of the patients maintained a sustained weight gain over the nine months of postoperative observation. However, the other four showed no consistent change of weight compared to pre-operative levels. This group included the two most severely underweight patients who had a pre-operative BMI of below 15.[119] Even the relative normalisation of weight in the two successfully treated patients came at the cost of an invasive procedure and a potential need to keep the electrodes in the brain for the rest of their lives (because nobody has conclusively ruled out that longstanding DBS produces addictive effects in its own right). The BBC online news headline of 7 March 2013, "Deep brain stimulation 'helps in severe anorexia nervosa'" (http://www.bbc.co.uk/news/health-21674836), was thus premature (as is often the case for media headlines on presumed medical "breakthroughs"). More evidence from larger studies with longer postoperative observation periods is needed to assess whether DBS really helps in anorexia and other eating disorders – with the proviso that ethical committees are prepared to approve further therapeutic studies of DBS in anorexia on the basis of these mixed data.

The editors of a recently published major textbook on neuromodulation techniques asked a number of experts for thoughts on *Neuromodulation for Emerging Applications*.[120] The "visionary" contributions cover applications of deep brain stimulation to obesity, blood pressure control, tinnitus, Alzheimer's disease and the minimally conscious state (MCS), although for most of these applications none or very little data from human DBS were available at the time of writing. The idea of treating obesity with DBS of the hypothalamus was based on a small study from the 1970s, when Danish neurosurgeons stimulated the lateral hypothalamus in overweight patients and elicited a hunger response in three out of five patients. In these patients they destroyed parts of the lateral hypothalamus and reported some transient decreases of calorie intake but no lasting weight changes. It is an interesting ethical question, which we will revisit in Chapter 4, whether such limited success of destructive surgery provides a sufficiently strong basis for experimental treatments that entail DBS of the same area.

For now, the state of psychiatric DBS and its public perception have been summarised succinctly by Marwan Hariz, Professor of Functional Neurosurgery at the National Hospital of Neurology and Neurosurgery in London:

> The introduction of the technique in psychiatry has generated much debate, and in the past decade far fewer patients have been treated than articles published.... However, the lay media have been almost unanimously positive, uncritically presenting deep brain stimulation as a high tech innovation with a promising future, echoing the reports of the lay press during the heyday of lobotomy, before the turn of the tide and demise of that procedure.[121]

3

The Brain Controls Itself: From Brain Reading to Brain Modulation via Neurofeedback

3.1 Biofeedback and therapy: the beginnings

Neal Miller, one of the pioneers of animal neurofeedback (see Chapter 1), always pursued his biofeedback work with clinical applications in mind. The opportunity to use physiological control training to modify psychiatric (and physical) disorders was met with great interest by the psychiatric community, which was only slowly moving beyond its psychoanalytic traditions. Throughout the 1970s and early 1980s EEG neurofeedback and biofeedback in general was approached with great optimism by basic and clinical researchers from a wide range of fields. A look at the table of contents of a volume on *Biofeedback and self control*, where Miller had assembled what he thought to be the most important papers of 1973/74 in this field, gives an idea of the number of applications where biofeedback was tried.[122] The sections on basic sciences covered "visceral learning", which included the control of heart rate and salivation, and two areas of neurofeedback, "evoked potentials and motor units" (in rats, cats and macaque monkeys) and "electroencephalographic control" (in humans). The clinical syndromes for which biofeedback was attempted included tension headache, high blood pressure, chronic anxiety and eating disorders. Even complex disturbances of the coordination of heart rhythms, such as the common syndrome of atrial fibrillation or the relatively rare Wolff Parkinson White (WPW) syndrome, were targeted with operant conditioning procedures. Neurofeedback protocols with EEG signals were being developed for epilepsy. The American neuroscientist Maurice Sterman, for example, trained epilepsy patients to increase activity in the 12 Hz–14 Hz frequency range. A successful increase in this sensorimotor rhythm was accompanied by a marked reduction in seizure frequency, an important clinical improvement. The problem with this though, as with many other neurofeedback studies, was that patient numbers were small (only six epilepsy patients participated) and there was no placebo control group. Sterman explained:

> The epileptics who have come to our program are seeking desperately to find a solution to their substantial medical problem. In at least one instance, an attempt to retain such a patient in our study for control procedures was not successful; the lack of positive results after several months lead to his withdrawal from the program. Efforts to explain the need for control data did not impress this individual.

The difficulty of recruiting sufficient numbers of patients to neuro-feedback studies, and particularly control patients who would undergo lengthy training without receiving much benefit, has remained a major obstacle to progress in this field. However, another study, on tension headache, did employ a full controlled design, with a placebo and a no-treatment group, although groups were small with six patients each. Researchers working with the American engineer and psychologist Thomas Budzynski used feedback of electrical activity from muscles rather than the brain. This is called EMG (electromyographic) biofeedback. Their basic setup consisted of a number of electrodes placed on the forehead which were connected to an amplifier. The muscle activity that was recorded was converted into an auditory signal. A higher rate of clicks corresponded to higher muscle activity, and patients were trained to downregulate the number of clicks. Patients received 16 training sessions of 30 minutes each over two months. In addition, they were asked to do two brief relaxation exercises per day at home. Patients charted their headaches on an hourly basis before, during and for three months after the intervention. Whereas the patients who received real EMG feedback managed to relax their frontal muscles after two or three sessions, the patients in the placebo group, who received the taped feedback from other patients, continued to show heightened muscle activity. The crucial finding was that only the group who received real feedback training showed clinical benefits in reduced headache levels, enabling them to reduce their dose of tranquillisers and painkillers. A few patients were contacted after 18 months and still reported reduced headaches. This study, albeit small, already contained all the elements of the protocol of a clinical biofeedback trial: control groups; homework to supplement the laboratory training; transfer sessions to assess whether patients maintained physiological control without feedback; long-term follow-up and information about real-life benefits, such as medication reduction. The investigators also offered patients in the placebo and no-treatment groups the option to receive the actual training after the completion of the trial, and most of them took it up. This is important from an ethical point of view; if a trial shows effects of the tested intervention, patients who were randomised to the control groups should also get an opportunity to receive it whenever possible.

These early trials on common health problems for which there was (and is) no satisfactory remedy, such as tension headaches, ushered in the development of a very active field of clinical biofeedback, mainly offered through physicians and psychologists in private practice in the United States. Research continued into the effects and mechanisms of neurofeedback, with a focus on the potential to control epileptic seizures. Ten years later, in 1983, Sterman provided an even more optimistic assessment of the clinical effects of EEG neurofeedback in epilepsy. His reading of the literature over the preceding ten years suggested "abundant confirmations of this therapeutic effect in man" and that questions of specificity had been "put to rest". He also reported on a new neurofeedback trial with epilepsy patients who had not responded well to anti-epileptic drugs. Patients played an EEG-controlled football game and scored goals by increasing the sensorimotor rhythm. After six weeks of training with three sessions per week, seizure rates declined significantly, and this effect was not observed in a placebo intervention, where the EEG recorded from other patients was used to control the football game.[123] The psychologist Joel F. Lubar from Tennessee also reported positive effects on epilepsy.[124] He estimated that by 1983 about 250 patients had been included in epilepsy biofeedback studies. One important observation of the early neurofeedback researchers was that when patients had experienced a reduction of their seizures and then the training was stopped, the frequency of the seizures could go up again. Similar effects can be seen after abrupt withdrawal of anti-epileptic drugs. Lubar therefore weaned the patients off the neurofeedback training very gradually, over a period of 50 days. Such rebound effects suggest that the neurofeedback procedure did, indeed, have specific effects on the symptoms but they also bring up the important ethical and safety issue of dependency that we have already encountered for DBS. If patients become dependent for symptom control on a continuous intervention the investigators who trial the procedure need to ensure that it is available in the long-term. Most clinical trials are conducted over weeks or months, not years and it is not clear who provides the intervention when the research funding ends.

3.2 Training elite musicians and surgeons

In the 1980s researchers also started using neurofeedback for cognitive enhancement.[125] Some of this work was based on observations of monkeys performing a short-term memory task. The monkeys had to memorise a visual cue on the right or left side and then press the appropriate button after an eight second blank interval. The researchers found that learning depended on the state of the monkeys' brains, which was recorded with implanted electrodes. Monkeys learnt this task much more rapidly if their frontal lobes were in a state of electrical negativity, which indicated activation of specific sets of inhibitory nerve cells.[125] Similar effects of improved learning or recognition of visual patterns after slow potential shifts were observed during EEG recordings in humans.[126] If particular electrical brain signatures and rhythms are associated with better performance, it is the logical next step to see whether their active modulation improves performance. Successful up-regulation of the sensorimotor rhythm, the beta frequency rhythm related to the "idling" activity of the motor cortex, indeed resulted in better scores on the continuous performance task (CPT).[127] In this task, participants have to press a key on a keyboard in response to a specific type of visual stimulus, but not to other, similar stimuli. Because of the similarity of the stimuli, these tasks can be difficult and are used in the psychological laboratory to assess a person's attention levels. A common problem with such laboratory tests is that they are often not particularly relevant to real-life situations. A person could be a top performer on the CPT and still overlook oncoming cars in real-life traffic situations. The next question therefore is whether neurofeedback can become relevant to skills required for everyday activities. This question was addressed in a series of fascinating studies with music students and other professionals who need high levels of motor skills. The investigators from London studied students from the Royal College of Music, one of the leading training centres for instrumental performance in the world. The students had to perform two pieces of their own choice before a panel of expert judges before and after five weeks of EEG neurofeedback training with two sessions per week. The judges, who were external to the college and did not know what training group the performers were in, rated the overall quality, musical understanding, stylistic accuracy and interpretive imagination of the young musicians. The students who trained to increase their theta over their alpha rhythms and thus shift their brain rhythms to lower frequencies did indeed improve on all the assessed scores. Of course, these effects may have been non-specific and relied mainly on improved relaxation and reduced stress levels, but even this would be useful for professional musicians. As musical lay people we tend to forget that even the most accomplished musicians suffer from stage fright. Famous examples include the pianists Franz Liszt, Vladimir Horowitz and Glenn Gould, and a survey of over 2,000 instrument players in London orchestras yielded a rate of 16% significant performance anxiety.[128]

The research group from London also tested whether dancing proficiency could be improved with biofeedback training. They recruited pairs of dancers from the ballroom and Latin dancing teams of their university who went through ten sessions of neurofeedback or biofeedback training to modulate heart rate variability. Two experts assessed their dance performance with rating scales familiar from shows such as *Strictly Come Dancing*, a popular dance competition on British TV. Both the neurofeedback and the biofeedback groups improved about half a point on a scale from one to five, which could be a decisive amount in such a competition.[129]

Even more spectacularly, the researchers from London trained budding ophthalmic surgeons with SMR neurofeedback and observed that they performed microsurgery better and faster after the intervention.[130] Again, these improvements could be put down to non-specific effects of improved concentration and it is not known whether simply practising the tasks in questions would create the same results. However, too much practice (certainly in music and sport but probably also in surgery) can have the opposite effect and even result in disabling conditions, such as cramps of the practising limb. Mental training strategies are therefore a standard component of elite performance training in music and sports, and enhancing it with direct brain modulation would be a fascinating prospect. It is currently hotly debated whether performance enhancement with drugs or external brain stimulation is ethically acceptable and safe. Surely, if similar effects can be obtained with self-regulation of the brain, this would make these decisions much easier because the person whose performance is enhanced remains in the driving seat and does not hand over control to a pharmaceutical company or an electromagnetic stimulator.

3.3   Clinical biofeedback today

Biofeedback interventions are now available from several thousand doctors, psychologists and other healthcare professionals worldwide. Three professional societies, the Association for Applied

Psychophysiology and Biofeedback (AAPB), the International Society for Neurofeedback & Research (ISNR) and the Biofeedback Foundation of Europe (BFE) promote the clinical use of these techniques and certify their practitioners. There are several international conferences per year, several textbooks covering the foundations and applications and at least two journals largely dedicated to bio- and neurofeedback (*Applied Psychophysiology and Biofeedback*, published by Springer, and *Journal of Neurotherapy*, published by Taylor and Francis). Biofeedback is on offer for a wide variety of neurological and psychiatric disorders, including addiction, anxiety, attention deficit/hyperactivity disorder (ADHD), depression and the classic target for neurofeedback, epilepsy. However, its applications also span the wider range of general medical conditions, including asthma, chronic pain syndromes, incontinence and high blood pressure. In the UK, biofeedback is not routinely available through the National Health Service, but in the USA and other countries some insurance plans reimburse its costs for some disorders. With this high level of professional organisation, the wide spectrum of targeted disorders and partial support from healthcare funders one would assume that there is good scientific evidence for the effectiveness of biofeedback. However, such evidence has been hard to establish for a variety of reasons.

Epilepsy is one of the disorders with the longest history of biofeedback interventions. We have already encountered the small but well-controlled studies conducted by Sterman in the 1970s and 1980s. Although computing power has increased and software has become more sophisticated the field has not moved on much since then. Clinical trials are still relatively small, and probably only a few hundred patients worldwide have been included over the last four decades. However, a high proportion experienced a significant reduction in the frequency of their seizures, often over 50%. Amongst the patients who responded were those with complex partial seizures. As we saw in Section 2.1, these patients suffer from periods of loss of consciousness, during which they can move around and engage in activities that observers often perceive as strange or repetitive. They also frequently experience hallucinations or other perceptual aberrations. These attacks can interfere in a major way with a person's everyday life, obviously making it impossible for them to drive, but can also affect their work and relationships and even result in criminal prosecution, depending on the nature of the automatic activities. Another danger arising from complex partial seizures is that they develop into life-threatening, generalised seizures. Although the last four decades have seen the introduction of many effective drugs to control such seizures (anticonvulsant or anti-epileptic drugs), a considerable number of patients do not become completely seizure free. In some treatment-refractory patients the seizures are so frequent and severe that they are considered for an operation, where the brain area responsible for generating the seizures is removed, as in the cases explored by Penfield (Section 2.3). This procedure requires lengthy monitoring, where electrodes are placed inside the patient's brain to locate the focus, and can have considerable side effects if the focus resides in areas supporting memory or other cognitive functions, which can be damaged during surgery. An alternative to drug therapy that may obviate the need for surgery should, therefore, be welcomed. However, in order to convince neurologists that neurofeedback is such an alternative and that it might work in patients where drugs have failed, larger trials would be needed. Sterman has pointed out that the usual sponsor of clinical trials, the pharmaceutical industry, is not particularly interested in neurofeedback, and this may be one of the reasons for the lack of large trials. Another reason for the slow take-up of neurofeedback in the epilepsy community may be that it is time-consuming for patients and, if combined with quantitative evaluation of abnormal EEG patterns, labour-intensive for clinicians. This lack of new data is disappointing because, at least in theory, EEG neurofeedback should be perfectly suited for the treatment of epilepsy, which is, after all, characterised by specific abnormal EEG patterns (unlike ADHD and the other psychiatric disorders that are targeted with EEG neurofeedback).

The biggest area of clinical neurofeedback today is probably its use on ADHD in children, which also has the largest evidence base. Over a thousand patients have so far been included in clinical trials.[131–134] These numbers are impressive because neurofeedback training requires many sessions in the laboratory or doctor's office, often 20 or 30 or more, over weeks or months. Children and their parents are nevertheless interested in this technique because ADHD can be very disruptive to a child's development and performance in school. Although the symptoms can often be well-controlled with stimulant drugs, such as methylphenidate (brand name Ritalin) these drugs do not work for everyone and can have side effects. Furthermore, there are increased concerns in wider society about the dramatic increase in stimulant prescriptions for children that has occurred over the last decade. The BBC report "Use of ADHD drugs 'increases by 50% in six years'" of 13 August 2013 (www.bbc.co.uk/news/health-23674235) is just one of a multitude of new items highlighting this, often controversial, debate.

Several clinical trials with neurofeedback in ADHD, targeting a variety of EEG parameters, have now been published that demonstrate superior effects to control interventions. It is not straightforward to design such a control intervention, and one option is to compare neurofeedback with attention training that does not use brain signals. Such attention training programmes also improve ADHD symptoms somewhat, and thus constitute a relatively conservative control (it is harder to demonstrate the effect of a new intervention against another effective treatment, but this is what is needed if one wants to introduce a technically more demanding – and more expensive – new treatment). It is encouraging that neurofeedback has effects over and above those of attention or concentration training that does not directly target the brain. One reason could be that neurofeedback modulates specific brain mechanisms that are abnormal in ADHD. This is not likely because the EEG of ADHD patients is not particularly abnormal and because a variety of different EEG protocols have been used to improve ADHD symptoms. Less specific effects of neural regulation, for example the general enabling effect of learning to control one's own brain, are more likely to underlie these positive clinical effects. There are several caveats, for example that improvements have not been dramatic (the children merely improved slightly on scales where parents assess their symptoms) and have certainly not obviated the need for medication. Furthermore, a recent meta-analysis (statistical analysis combining all available clinical trials) of non-pharmacological interventions for ADHD[135] has concluded that the superiority of neurofeedback over placebo is not statistically significant if only trials using blinded assessments (where the rater is not aware of the patient's treatment condition) are included in the analysis.

In the UK, the most recent appraisal of interventions for ADHD by the Royal College of Psychiatrists and the British Psychological Society (from 2009) concluded that biofeedback "is probably not used as a significant intervention in UK clinical practice."[136] However, in countries with a larger proportion of private or privately commissioned medicine, such as the USA, Germany, the Netherlands or Switzerland, EEG neurofeedback for ADHD is more widely available.

At present the main standard components of interventions for children with ADHD are training sessions with the parents and, if these are unsuccessful, stimulant drugs. Particularly for children who (or whose parents) are reluctant to use stimulants, neurofeedback might become another option to try before long-term drug treatment is considered. Once the software for real-time data analysis and feedback has been developed, EEG neurofeedback is not technically challenging. For example, it may only use the recording from one electrode, placed over the centre of the brain (called electrode Cz). This has made it possible to develop relatively cheap devices for home treatment, which are now on the market. Feedback-based training devices (for example based on gaming consoles) have already conquered people's homes in industrialised countries. Even neurofeedback has entered the market for video games. One example are the games developed by the NASA spinoff company SmartBrain (www.smartbraintech.com). EEG-based neurofeedback is being marketed for home training by Emotiv (www.emotiv.com). It is conceivable that parents will try to use a variety of these computerised training systems to improve their children's ADHD symptoms, regardless of the outcome of future clinical trials. This may be a general characteristic of medicine in the digital age. Patients (or their carers) may shop around the internet for solutions to medical problems to which the established professionals have no or only partial answers and try new technologies for themselves. This market is also much harder to regulate than that for prescription drugs because there is such widespread non-medical use of computer games. These new developments can have both positive and negative aspects. In our example of neurofeedback for ADHD, widespread home use coupled with online-assessments may actually produce patient numbers for clinical trials that are otherwise unattainable. On the negative side, uncontrolled use of computer training devices, including neurofeedback, may contribute to an overuse of computers and the internet, which is emerging as a new health problem in its own right.[137]

3.4   Neurofeedback: deep brain stimulation without surgery?

There is no doubt that electrical stimulation of specific brain areas can alter mental states and behaviour, not only in birds and rodents but also in primates, including humans. There is also considerable evidence that it can improve the symptoms of neurological and psychiatric disorders, at least in selected patient groups. One important downside is that it makes patients dependent on the stimulation device. Unlike lesion surgery, which changes the state of the brain once and for all, DBS only works as long as the stimulator is on. Earlier attempts to improve psychiatric conditions just with temporary stimulation (see Heath's programme described in Section 2.3) have not been successful. Because modern electrodes do not wear off too soon and the batteries can last for years and then be replaced, continuous stimulation is not a major practical problem for most patients (although it is too early to tell for the relatively recent use of DBS in psychiatry how many years the stimulation remains effective for). However, they may be uneasy about continuing dependence on a technical device. Dependence may also develop quite literally, in the sense of addiction. We saw in Section 2.3 that the rats in Olds's laboratory preferred the electrical stimulation of specific brain areas over other types of rewards and went through great efforts to obtain it, even accepting adverse and potentially dangerous consequences. These are all characteristic features of human addiction, and we cannot rule out that patients may also become addicted to deep brain stimulation, albeit less dramatically than Olds's rodents. Little is known about this because it is, of course, ethically unacceptable to perform experiments with the aim of making humans addicted to brain stimulation. However, it is likely that nerve cells in DBS patients will adjust to long-term stimulation, for example by changing their spontaneous firing patterns or by making different proteins. In this way they can form cellular "memories" of the stimulation. As a result, the chronic brain stimulation may become very much a part of the patient's normal neural network activity. This may also explain why patients do not like it when the stimulation is suddenly stopped. This is a common method for proving the clinical effects of DBS, to compare the patient's well-being between periods when the stimulator is on or off. After 6 or 12 months of DBS for OCD or depression many patients will report a deterioration of their mood and other symptoms if the stimulator is switched off for a while. However, whether the reason for this is that they have become dependent on the electrical stimuli or whether it reflects a genuine therapeutic effect of DBS is difficult to tell. After all, we would not say that alcohol cures depression (quite the contrary) just because a patient's mood deteriorates during an alcohol withdrawal.

Considering the technical, and possibly even physical, dependency involved in DBS, it would be an attractive option if patients could attain the same effects by self-regulating their brain activity. This opens up the possibility of reviving the clinical use of neurofeedback. One of the limitations of EEG-based neurofeedback was that it had low spatial precision. With EEG signals that are recorded from the scalp it is always very difficult to say where in the brain they are generated. Might functional MRI be an alternative? We have already encountered this technique for mapping out brain areas when discussing techniques for brain communication in Chapter 1. Compared to EEG it has the advantage that it localises brain signals to specific areas at a resolution of millimetres. The human brain has a volume of about one litre (equals one million cubic millimetres) and, with its resolution of approximately one millimetre, fMRI can thus potentially pick up signals from one million different places in the brain. Any one of them (and their interplay) could be crucial for a particular illness. Although this is still very far from the number of nerve cells in the human brain (100,000 million), it opens up a potential avenue for mapping out neural correlates of particular symptoms and trying to influence them (and the symptoms) with neurofeedback.

In order to understand how this might work, let us consider again the example of the motor control areas that are being used in basic forms of brain communication (Sections 1.6–1.8). fMRI-based brain communication is based on the observation that certain areas of the brain, such as the primary motor cortex, are activated not only while we are moving some part of our body, but also when we just imagine doing so. These activations differ according to the body parts involved in the movement. In the simplest case, we can observe higher activation in the left motor cortex when imagining moving the right arm, and higher activation in the right motor cortex when imagining moving the left arm. We discussed that this differential activation can be used to build a simple communication device to say "yes" (left motor cortex active) or "no" (right motor cortex active).

We can use the same idea to train the person in the scanner to up-regulate a specific part of their motor cortex. For example, if we show them feedback about the activation level in the area responsible for moving the right hand in the left motor cortex and ask them to drive it up they can do this by imagining or planning movements involving the right hand. Because it would be easy to do so with actual movements we would instruct them to do this without moving the hand (and can control this by attaching electrodes to their hands that would pick up activation of the hand muscles).

Feedback on brain activity levels can be given in a variety of ways. Visual feedback, such as the thermometer bar shown in Figure 3.1, is most commonly used, but one could also use tones of different pitches or tactile stimuli of varying pressure. The patient can now read from the feedback whether his/her strategy to drive up the area in question is successful. If the bar fails to go up they can adjust their strategy. For example, if they are told that they are getting feedback from the motor cortex but not from which exact area they may start by imagining hand movements and then try other body parts until they finally settle for imaginary kicks at a football because the feedback corresponds to activation of the foot area.

What could be the use of training people to up-regulate specific parts of their motor cortex in this way? It could be used to enhance the precision of BCI communication for the paralysed. Another application would be

Real-time fMRI neurofeedback setup

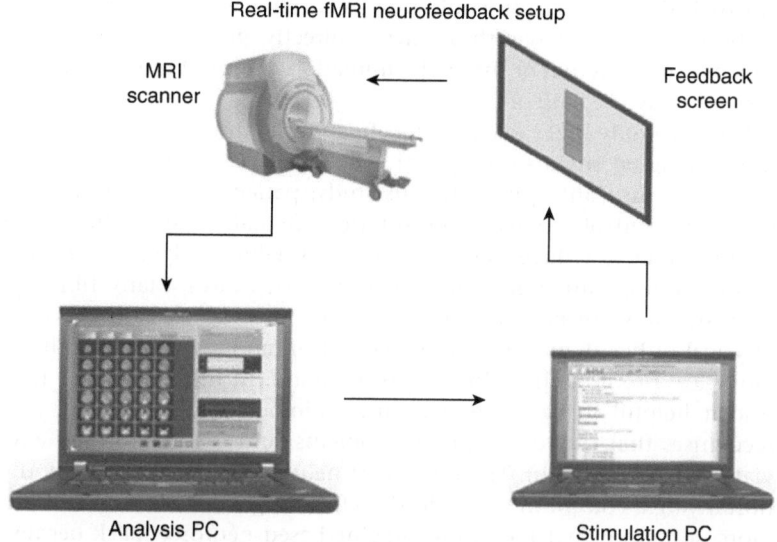

Figure 3.1   The components of a neurofeedback laboratory. Brain data are acquired in the MRI scanner and transferred in real-time to an analysis computer, where they are also analysed in real-time (for example one frame every two seconds). This corresponds to the feature extraction phase of the BCI (Section 1.6). A translation algorithm then converts the extracted feature of the MRI signal into a command for a feedback signal, which can be displayed to the participant while he or she is in the scanner

motor training in sports or music. Both fields make increasing use of mental practice, and the effects of EEG neurofeedback in music students and dancers have been encouraging. Mental practice can increase the precision of motor programmes and avoids injuries from overuse. One problem with mental practice or any mental imagery is that it is very difficult to control. How do the trainer, and indeed the trained, know that mental imagery was performed successfully? This can be controlled through measuring brain activation. What is more, with the neurofeedback procedure the musician or athlete could actually adjust their imagery strategies to attain the optimum level of brain activation.

Can this new approach through high resolution functional imaging also help to revitalise the clinical applications of neurofeedback? The 20 years of research with functional MRI have resulted in a detailed understanding of many of the brain circuits supporting perception, thought, action and emotion, and efforts have also been made to map out their dysfunctions. It would now be attractive to utilise this information in order to target these circuits directly, but this time not with DBS or other external or internal stimulation devices, but through self-regulation by the patients.

The first study that looked at the effects of neurofeedback with functional imaging signals on clinical symptoms was published in 2005 by a group in California.[138] In this study, patients with fibromyalgia trained to control activity in the anterior cingulate gyrus of the frontal lobe in order to reduce their levels of pain. Fibromyalgia is a chronic and disabling pain syndrome with unknown causes. Many fibromyalgia sufferers are keen to emphasise that they are suffering from a physical rather than a psychiatric condition and are confident that a biological proof of their illness can be found. In this quest they may find it helpful to be presented with a biological illness model that recognises that the roots of their problems, and the key to their alleviation, is in the brain. The take-up of neurofeedback methods by the fibromyalgia community should therefore be good. Pain was, furthermore, a natural first target for imaging-based neurofeedback because the pathways of pain processing in the human brain are relatively well known. In addition to the primary sensory cortex, which receives the incoming tactile signals from the receptors in the skin (with a few relay stations in between), they comprise areas of affective processing in the limbic system, for example the amygdala, and in the cingulate cortex. The cingulate cortex functions as an intermediary between the limbic areas, involved in emotion and memory, and areas in the prefrontal cortex for thought and planning. It is an ideal target for neurofeedback because it is one of the areas potentially under conscious control but at the same time able to modulate the affective responses that contribute crucially to our experience of pain. Indeed, the investigators found that those patients who learnt to control activity in the anterior part of the cingulate gyrus (ACC) were more able to control their pain and rated their pain as lower after the training session. Because chronic pain syndromes are very difficult to manage, these promising results received international media coverage. However, further trials of the longer-term effects of this intervention in patients with chronic pain have been disappointing. Although this has dampened the enthusiasm of researchers working in this area, pain control seems to be one of the more obvious targets for clinical applications of fMRI-based neurofeedback (fMRI-NF). After all, EEG-based neurofeedback, which operates at a much lower spatial resolution, had some success in the control of tension headaches and other pain syndromes.

3.5 Neurofeedback: psychotherapy without therapist?

Moving from chronic pain to potential psychiatric applications of fMRI-based neurofeedback, one might wonder whether similar results to those obtained by DBS in depression could be obtained with the neurofeedback method. One reservation about DBS and other stimulation techniques in depression is that patients essentially play a passive role and are controlled by their doctors, rather than exercising control themselves. The influential self-efficacy model developed by the American social psychologist Albert Bandura posits that depression is sustained by an increasing loss of the sense of control of oneself and the environment. According to Bandura:[139]

> People have to live with a psychic environment that is largely of their own making. Many human distresses result from failures to control disturbing, ruminative thoughts. Control of one's thought processes is therefore a key factor in self-regulation of emotional states.

Our research group thus set itself the challenge to design a neurofeedback protocol for patients with depression. Initially, we had planned to target the same area as used for the first DBS study, the subgenual anterior cingulate cortex, but it turned out that down-regulation of a brain area is much harder to achieve than up-regulation. This seems to be common sense; we have a very long list of different mental activities at our disposal that we can use to try and up-regulate a brain area, but we are much more limited in what we can take away from whatever we are engaged in at any moment. It also seemed that with a fixed target area we would forego one of the big attractions of imaging-based neurofeedback, that it can be flexibly adjusted to whatever situation an individual patient finds themselves in. One of the reasons that we are all different in our emotional experience is that different brain processes are involved in different people (and the experience that everyone's mood fluctuates would even suggest that there is further variation over time). It therefore seemed a good idea to locate our neurofeedback targets individually patient by patient, and session by session. To this end, we used a localiser scan, where we showed patients emotionally charged pictures. In order to bring out the networks involved in responses to pleasant stimuli, we contrasted positive (for example, nice food, serene scenery) with negative pictures (for example, scenes of human suffering, gloomy landscapes). The positive emotion network was then used as the target for neurofeedback and patients were trained

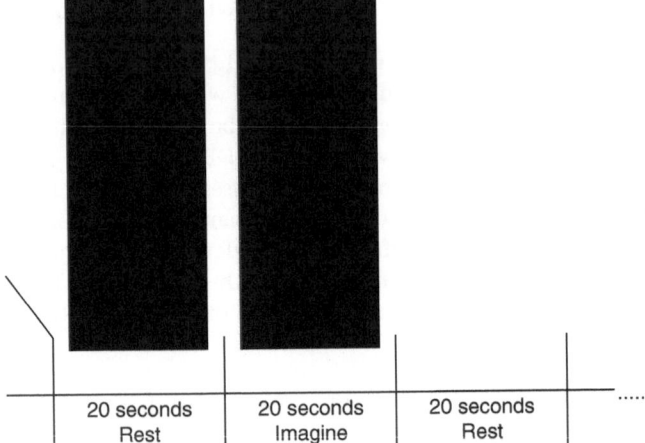

Figure 3.2   Alternation of rest and up-regulation/mental imagery blocks in a typical fMRI-neurofeedback protocol

Source: From a study on neurofeedback in Parkinson's disease by Subramanian and colleagues.[140]

to drive its activity up during 20-second periods, alternating with 20-second periods of rest. Overall, they did this for 20 minutes each in four weekly sessions (Figure 3.2).

We tested eight patients, all with a long-standing history of depression. What was interesting is that they all seemed to enjoy the procedure and managed to control their emotion networks rather well. The only clue we had given them is that we were targeting the areas that we had localised with the emotional pictures. The obvious strategy for up-regulation during the neurofeedback sessions was to try imaging the pictures they had just seen, which is what most of the patients did. However, they soon found that it actually worked better to try and evoke positive images that related to themselves, for example memories of happy events. We thus managed to engage them with positive aspects of their own lives, which they had almost forgotten. Some of them described the process as psychotherapy without a therapist!

The clinical effects of our depression study were also encouraging.[141] The patients in the neurofeedback group improved by about 30% on their symptom score over the one-month trial, whereas a control group, who performed emotional imagery for the same duration outside the scanner, did not improve at all (Figure 3.3).

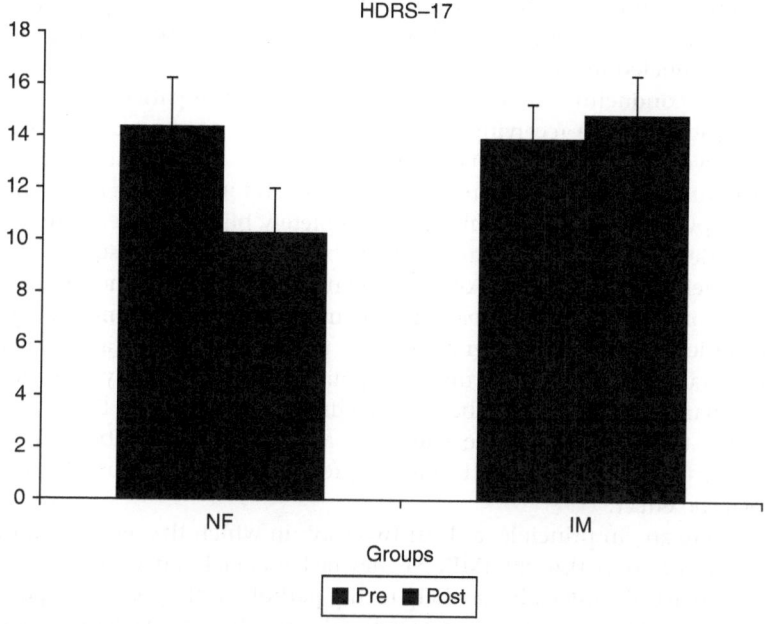

Figure 3.3 Improvement of symptoms of depression after fMRI-NF in pilot study

Note: The Hamilton Depression Rating Scale (HDRS) assesses depressive symptoms with 17 items, looking at issues such as guilty feelings, suicidal thoughts, sleep, anxiety, appetite and sexual function. A score of seven or less generally denotes remission from depression. Symptom improvement occurred only in the neurofeedback (NF) group, but not in the imagery (IM) group. Reprinted from our neurofeedback study in depression.[141]

Does this mean that neurofeedback will be a new, risk-free treatment for depression? Before making any claims of this sort its short- and long-term benefits for patients with depression will have to be tested in rigorous trials. Essentially, the same standards apply as those required before the introduction of a new drug. We can be relatively certain that neurofeedback has no major direct side effects[142] but cannot rule out that some patients may experience parts of the procedure as stressful. Furthermore, we will have to show that the clinical benefits are not merely placebo effects induced by a patient's expectations (an automatic effect of being part of an intervention study) but that they are genuinely superior to those of other interventions.

The design of appropriate control conditions for clinical trials of neurofeedback is a challenge, though. The current standards of randomised controlled trials were developed with drug studies in mind, where the aim is to distinguish the chemical effects of a drug from the associated expectations. One of the principles of these trials is that they are conducted in a double blind fashion, which means that neither the person conducting the clinical assessments nor the patient are aware whether they are receiving the actual treatment or the placebo drug. However, when treatments require the active collaboration of the patient, which is the case in neurofeedback (and in all forms of psycho-therapy), these patients cannot be completely blind. Furthermore, the experience of gaining control over the brain, the increased self-efficacy and heightened awareness of one's mental state may all be non-specific components of neurofeedback that contribute to improvement across disorders. Although we can control for them with sophisticated exper-imental designs this may miss the point because these psychological mechanisms may actually be valuable drivers of change for the patient rather than a mere placebo effect. We also have to remember that an estimated 80% of the effect of antidepressant drugs is attributable to a placebo effect.

There are, in principle, at least two ways in which the self-regulation of brain activity through fMRI-NF may be beneficial in neurological and psychiatric disorders. It may help rectify pathological hyper- or hypoac-tivation of specific brain areas or networks. For this approach one would ideally identify the targeted pathological activation patterns in indi-vidual patients. Alternatively, neurofeedback may be used to boost the recruitment of compensatory circuits for particular tasks (e.g. motor control) or cognitive processes (e.g. emotion regulation). The latter possibility is particularly attractive in cases where brain tissue may have been damaged by the disease, for example in strokes, or where no clear abnormalities have been established, as in most psychiatric disorders. The 20 years of fMRI research have produced a wealth of information about the neural circuits underlying emotion and cognition. Based on patients' functional deficits we can assume that giving them control over these circuits may improve clinical symptoms. One example is emotion regulation, which is impaired in patients with affective disor-ders. If patients gain control over the neural circuits supporting emotion regulation it is likely that they will also gain control over the emotions themselves, which is a key target of depression therapy. The target areas for this approach are mainly in the frontal lobe (see Figure 3.4). Another approach starts from the observation that many patients with depres-sion are impaired in their ability to react to rewards or generally to have positive experiences (lack of enjoyment, anhedonia). It has been well-established through functional imaging in humans and a long tradition

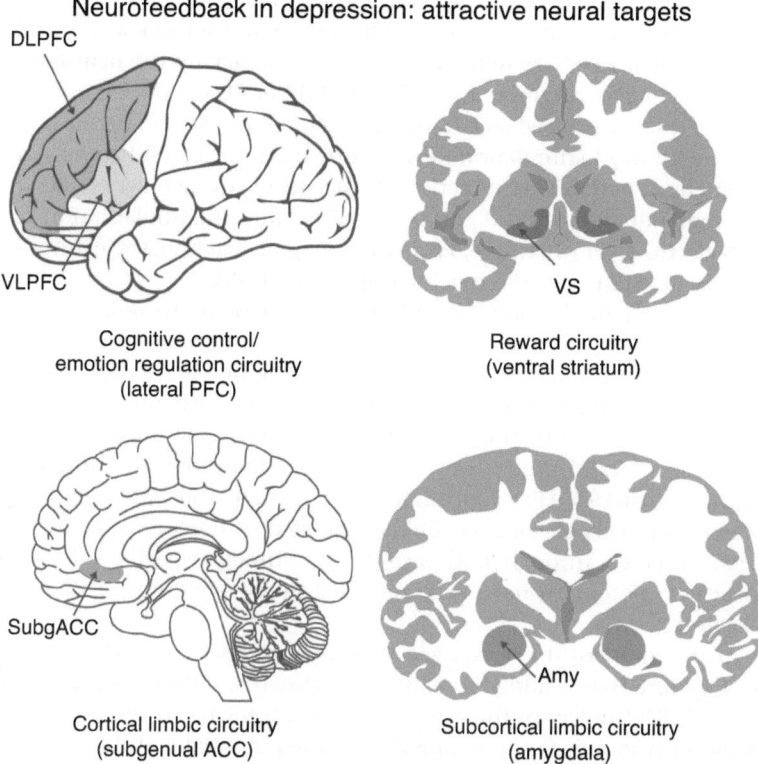

Figure 3.4   Areas and circuits that could be targeted by neurofeedback for depression. Reprinted from Esmail & Linden, 2012[143] with kind permission of Nova Science Publishers

of animal experiments that areas in the midbrain, striatum and frontal cortex, linked through the neurotransmitter dopamine, support the ability to experience and learn from rewards. These reward circuits would therefore be as attractive a target for fMRI-NF, as they are for DBS (Section 2.11).

In the future it may also become possible to combine neurofeedback and DBS in several ways. The placement of DBS electrodes and the selection of the exact stimulation protocol could be preceded by a phase of neurofeedback training. During this phase the patient could practice self-regulation of different brain areas and physicians could select for the subsequent brain stimulation those areas where the most promising clinical effects are observed. Another way of combining the two approaches might be through establishing neurofeedback as a transfer technology for DBS. Here the idea would be to pick up the neurophysiological changes produced by DBS with fMRI or EEG and then use these as targets for neurofeedback training. Although it is safe to perform MRI scans with most stimulation devices (one has to be careful about ferromagnetic materials and induction of currents in strong magnetic fields), the signal quality of fMRI can be impaired after the implantation of a DBS electrode. Furthermore, EEG is a more practical transfer technology because it is portable and much cheaper than fMRI.

Thus, it might become possible to teach patients to reproduce the effects of DBS by neurofeedback training and then explant the electrode again, avoiding long-term dependence on the device. If the effects of DBS can be mimicked by neurofeedback this may also aid the development of brain modulation protocols for patients who are not suitable for DBS or would prefer a self-regulation training over the implantation of electrodes. However, slightly surprisingly, thus far no clear cut correlates of DBS effects that could be targeted with neurofeedback have been observed through EEG recordings, although specific effects on local field potentials have been recorded invasively during DBS in PD (Section 2.5).

At the moment it is envisaged that neurofeedback, like DBS, will be a procedure that is added to existing treatments, rather than replacing them. With this caveat the prospect of neurofeedback as a treatment for depression sounds far more prosaic, but the potential is still huge. After all, about 10% of the world's population suffer from serious depression at least once in their lives, and about 30% of sufferers do not respond to existing therapies. This problem is unlikely to go away. In fact, if anything, depression seems to be on the increase worldwide and is recognised as one of the main reasons for chronic disability in industrialised countries. Any new treatment, even if it only provides partial recovery for a small subgroup of patients, would therefore have a huge impact on patients' well-being and healthcare costs.

3.6   Can neurofeedback improve Parkinson's disease?

If mental disorders are generally on the increase, this is true even more dramatically for diseases that are caused by a degeneration of the brain. With medical progress, life expectancy is continuing to increase. For example, there are currently three million people over 80 in the UK, and this number is expected to double by 2030! However, therapeutic progress in neurodegenerative disorders has not kept pace with that in other fields of medicine and the higher numbers of older people will therefore mean that more and more people will suffer from Alzheimer's, Parkinson's and other age-related disorders. New cures and treatments that stop disease progression, or at least improve everyday functioning, are sorely needed. Might neurofeedback come in here? Because we do not (yet) know how neurofeedback works we cannot say whether it may help to stop loss of nerve cells, or even promote growth of new ones. But we can start with a less ambitious project and see whether it helps patients with Parkinson's disease with their everyday functioning and to live independently for longer.

We can try and see, for example, whether neurofeedback will help John (not his real name), who was diagnosed with PD in 2005 at the age of 48. He had already stopped work as a civil engineer two years before the diagnosis was made because of his tremors. When he visited our research team in 2009 he was treated with the drugs pramipexole and rasagiline and his symptoms were predominantly tremors of the left hand and of the eyelids. This is a standard combination for early phases of PD. Pramipexole is a dopamine agonist, which means that it stimulates dopamine receptors even when dopamine is lacking, and thus restores some of the lost motor functions. Rasagiline has another mechanism of action; it blocks one of the enzymes that degrade dopamine and thus increases the levels of the remaining dopamine in the patient's brain. Both drugs are generally well tolerated, but one of his concerns was that he developed swelling of his legs. This is a relatively common side effect of pramipexole and of other anti-PD drugs so switching drugs was not really an option. He thought about reducing it, but then would that result in a worsening of his symptoms, for example making it impossible for him to drive?

At that time we had just developed a protocol for neurofeedback in PD. We knew that motor areas were good targets for up-regulation training from our experience with healthy individuals. We had also learnt that dysfunction of the supplementary motor area, one of the motor control areas in the frontal lobe, may be very relevant in PD.[144] We therefore started a small trial where patients learnt to up-regulate the supplementary motor area over two scanning sessions, without any overt movements but with mental strategies alone. The sessions were separated by two months, but we asked patients to practice their mental strategies for a few minutes on a daily basis. John was one of the first patients recruited to this study and this is how he described his experience:

Then I took part in the neurofeedback experiment at Bangor University. An experience which changed my whole approach to coping with PD. During the course of the various tests I discovered that when I thought about moving my arm it would become physically fatigued just as if I were moving it for real! I found that the harder I visualized movement the more real the effect. ... I decided to try improving my capacity to move my arm just by imagining it. Subsequently I found that after a week of mentally thinking through the task I was able to bend straight down and pick up a small coin from the floor. I have applied the neurofeedback technique to everything I do now. This had has a very positive effect on my symptoms. ... The high point of this for me was in February, when I was on an outing with people from my Welsh Learners group. One chap came over to reintroduce himself (I hadn't seen him in a year) and said "I thought you told me you had Parkinsons?" To which I replied, "That's right I did", "well where then ... it doesn't show!" ... I am now taking a lower dose of pramipexole and am feeling better than I did before taking part in the MRI scan programme last year. Oh and I recently managed to re-cover a garden shed roof, something I wouldn't have tackled a year ago.

For John the neurofeedback training had the desired effect of allowing him to reduce the dose of his medication. Perhaps even more importantly, the mental training gave him the confidence to tackle complex motor tasks that he had not performed since the onset of the disease. Although these may seem small steps and certainly do not amount to a cure of Parkinson's, they can make a difference to patients who otherwise face a relentless progression of their illness. The other four patients who took part in this first small trial at Bangor University in North Wales also improved. We used a standard test of motor functions in Parkinson's, the UPDRS (Unified Parkinson's Disease Rating Scale). This test assesses the core motor domains commonly affected in Parkinson's, posture, gait, tremor, muscle rigidity and slowing of movements. All patients improved on this scale, but not everyone improved in all domains. John, for example, mainly improved in his ability to control his posture and to move fluently. Perhaps this depended on the strategies they had used to up-regulate their motor cortex. All patients seemed to enjoy the experience and were interested in coming back for more sessions.

When we discussed the depression study we were concerned about the placebo effect. Do we need to worry about this here, too? Might the improvement be caused by patient expectation that they ought to improve under a new intervention rather than any true effect of the treatment? Alternatively, do we not have to worry about this because placebo effects are less relevant to neurodegenerative disorders like Parkinson's disease than to psychiatric disorders like depression? This last is certainly not the case. Placebo effects can make a major contribution to drug responses in Parkinson's disease. One study even demonstrated that patients who received a placebo drug instead of levodopa still responded with a release of dopamine in their basal ganglia![145] Comparison with control groups is therefore as important in Parkinson's disease as it is in depression. We tested the specificity of the neurofeedback effect by comparing our five patients with five others with equally severe Parkinson's symptoms who also went into the fMRI scanner and received the same instructions to engage in mental motor imagery, but did not receive any feedback about their brain activity. This group did not improve.[140] This is a first indication that it is not just the mental training but the feedback about its effects on the brain and the specific brain regulation training that yielded the clinical benefit.

However, it will be difficult to rule out the effects of expectancy and motivation completely in the bigger studies that are now necessary. Lack of motivation is part of the syndrome of Parkinson's and contributes to the motor problems. If we dismissed as just a placebo effect every intervention that "merely" improved motivation and gave patients an expectation of improvement, we may restrict the development of new interventions too much. The most practically relevant question will be whether neurofeedback works better than other training programmes that use less expensive and more widely available equipment. For example, at Cardiff University we are currently comparing a neurofeedback-based intervention for Parkinsons's disease with exercise on a gaming console. If training with a gaming console produces the same results as neurofeedback, this would be a very cost effective alternative. But even if physical exercise on its own does not work, it may still become a very attractive tool to help patients transfer the motor planning strategies they learn during neurofeedback into daily exercises using these widely available devices for home use.

3.7 Neurofeedback and neurorehabilitation

Many brain disorders result in irreversible damage to certain brain structures. A common example is a stroke, where a lack of blood flow – and consequently lack of oxygen – leads to the death of neurons. The immediate symptoms correspond to the function of the lost area. For example, if the stroke affected one of the language areas, which are located in the left hemisphere in most people, the patient would suffer from aphasia, a difficulty in understanding or producing speech. If the stroke affected the left motor cortex or its connections to the spinal cord, the main symptom might be weakness or complete paralysis of the right arm or leg. However, such loss of speech or motor functions can be partly reversed even if the damage to brain tissue is permanent. With the aid of rehabilitation specialists, such as physiotherapists or speech and language therapists, patients can often recover some of their lost functions. The underlying mechanisms in the brain are not very well understood, but it is thought that plasticity plays a major role. Neural plasticity denotes the ability of nerve cells to form new connections and thus take over new functions. Although the brain's plasticity is at its most impressive during childhood and early adolescence, such compensatory mechanisms have been demonstrated even in the aging brain. This may explain the partial recovery of functions that occurs spontaneously in many patients after a stroke or other brain injury. The philosophy behind neurorehabilitation is that it enhances this neural plasticity with specific exercises. The neural theory behind this goes back to Canadian psychologist Donald Hebb, whose postulate that "neurons that fire together wire together" we encountered in Section 1.5. Thus, if we can stimulate certain neurons to fire in conjunction with specific physical or mental exercises, we may be able to induce them to form new connections that can support sustained compensation for the lost functions. With this theoretical background in mind, direct neural training through neurofeedback should be an attractive tool for such neurorehabilitation programmes.

This exciting possibility – to use neurofeedback in the rehabilitation of patients with stroke or other focal brain damage – has so far not been explored in formal clinical studies, although the community of neurorehabilitation clinicians and engineers is increasingly becoming aware of this method. For example, in 2012 the department of neurorehabilitation engineering at the Swiss Federal Institute of Technology hosted the first international conference on clinical applications of neurofeedback. Rehabilitation engineers develop sophisticated electronic devices for the functional assessment of patients with brain injuries and other neurological disorders. For example, a team in Zurich has developed a kind of watch that monitors the activity levels of patients over weeks and months. Such devices have to be small and light and have to contain very durable batteries, which is a particular challenge. They can be extremely useful for the objective evaluation of the activity of stroke patients and thus help to measure whether rehabilitation programmes actually work, and especially if they work when patients have left inpatient rehabilitation and have to maintain their levels of activity at home. Although a stroke can leave patients permanently disabled, there are also many cases with excellent outcomes, for example almost complete restoration of function in a limb that had been paralysed initially. Engineers have also developed robots as aids for motor rehabilitation, to complement physiotherapy. For example, robots can move limbs passively in a very controlled fashion and apply sensory stimulation, which may be a first step in the recovery of motor functions. They can also be used to train patients to move against a force and to overcome disturbances of the movement path. Perhaps most importantly robots and other sensing devices, such as the balance boards available with gaming consoles, can provide very accurate feedback about a patient's movements and limb position and thus guide motor training. It thus makes perfect sense to include robots in rehabilitation after a stroke and other brain damage and the first trials that formally test this approach are under way. But one important limitation is that classic rehabilitation, including robotics, does not directly target the brain. It is also still very rare for investigators to obtain functional brain imaging measures before and after rehabilitation in order to ascertain the mechanisms of any changes, and whether they were really supported by Hebbian plasticity. The reasons are the high cost of brain scans and the attitude of many clinicians who would be content to have an intervention that works even if its exact mechanisms of action are unknown. Neurofeedback has the attraction of providing both, potentially identifying the areas that are crucial for plastic changes in the brain, and targeting these areas directly through self-regulation training. This is the main reason why clinicians, neuroscientists and engineers are currently getting very interested in the use of neurofeedback in neurorehabilitation.

Neurofeedback can provide direct access to the patient's brain, then the engineers can construe training devices for the transfer of neurofeedback strategies into real-life. Stroke would be a good target for neurofeedback because the changes that have to occur in the brain for a recovery of motor functions to take place are relatively well known. The mechanisms of plasticity in stroke have been studied over many decades in animal models, and over the past 30 years with imaging studies in patients. For example, fMRI has shown that corresponding areas in the unaffected hemisphere are recruited to regain motor functions or speech. Another technique for studying the mechanisms of stroke recovery is transcranial magnetic stimulation (TMS), where electrical fields in the brain are changed by applying strong magnetic fields over the scalp. This can enhance or interfere with neural processes and thus help identify those that are functionally relevant for a particular motor skill. This method has revealed that areas around the lesion inhibit the surviving neurons within the affected area in the acute stages of stroke. Stroke rehabilitation seems to work through reducing this local inhibition and by promoting integration across hemispheres, but physiotherapists and engineers on the ground do not know whether and how they are changing an individual patient's brain circuits in the desired direction. This is where fMRI and neurofeedback can come in to provide regular snapshots of the functional activation of motor or language networks and to train these networks directly.

In terms of its potential impact on public health, neurofeedback operates at the other end of the spectrum compared to the brain computer interfaces for communication and robot control we discussed in Chapter 1. The latter devices require very long-term training and also invasive implantation of electrode grids and their main scope is in patients with complete paralysis after brainstem stroke or motor neuron disease. These techniques could make all the difference to a small number of people. Conversely, neurofeedback will probably always be a small cog in the complex machine of therapies, but its great flexibility means that it can potentially be applied to a wide range of neurological and psychiatric disorders and confer a small benefit to many patients. Mental and neurodegenerative disorders have already become the most important public health problem in industrialised countries, in terms of the numbers of people affected and the reduction in their quality of life, and we have no causal cures to stop the progression. Even small improvements to patients' lives, which may allow them to stay in work longer, take up their hobbies again, or spend less time in hospital, can therefore make a real difference for both patients and society.

Neurofeedback and behaviour

Many mental and behavioural disorders are characterised by pathological reactions to certain cues. For example, in patients suffering from post-traumatic stress disorder after a major traffic accident, even the distant sound of an ambulance can trigger intense fear. Another example is addiction, where small doses of the substance, or even associated sensory cues (for example, a picture of the favourite drink), can trigger a relapse. These abnormal behavioural responses have a correlate in the brain reward systems. In people with substance addiction the ventral striatum and other areas of the reward pathways are hyperactive during exposure to drug-related cues, for example pictures of drink, cigarette fumes or lines of cocaine. If we can identify these craving-related brain responses with fMRI it should also be possible to target them with neurofeedback. The basic idea is to train patients to downregulate the hyperactive areas and networks while they are exposed to the drug-related cues. It should be possible to develop such protocols for any substance addiction and any other disorder where specific cues and brain systems can be identified. Anxiety disorders, such as specific phobias, come to mind, where patients could be trained to downregulate a hyperactive amygdala during exposure to spiders or other aversive stimuli. Another potential example would be OCD, where patients could be trained to downregulate hyperactive circuits between the frontal lobe and the basal ganglia while being exposed to contaminated objects. The concept is the same as that underlying surgery or DBS, but whereas cingulotomy or capsulotomy destroy pathways between basal ganglia and the frontal lobe and DBS permanently modifies their activity, stimulus-coupled neurofeedback would merely modulate them when the risk of developing symptoms and dysfunctional behaviours is highest, which may enhance the efficacy of the brain modulation and help reduce side effects.

Neurofeedback on a smartphone?

Some of the early DBS work also tried to influence a person's behaviour by pairing certain stimuli or behaviours with pleasant electrical stimulation. Such direct conditioning is not an option in current clinical DBS approaches because they do not involve stimulation of hedonic areas. However, it is conceivable that DBS for certain behavioural disorders will be enhanced by pairing the stimulation with particular cues, or changing the stimulation parameters dependent on the patient's behaviour. The next step in the development of DBS for movement disorders will be to devise, so-called, closed loop systems, where the stimulation parameters adapt to the state of the brain, for example the neurophysiological signals picked up locally in the subthalamic nucleus.[146] Such a closed loop can also receive input from an external sensing device. For example, the delivery of inhibitory stimuli to reward centres could be increased whenever a person's smartphone detects that the patient is approaching their local pub. Similarly, if cue-related neurofeedback, as outlined in the previous section, is successful in reducing cravings, patients could use the mental strategies learnt in the fMRI laboratory to control their behaviour in everyday situations.

A few sessions in the scanner would probably not be sufficient to sustain neurofeedback learning effects in the long-term. At some point the feedback training will need to be transferred to technologies that can be used in patients' homes or even whilst on the move. Amongst the brain recording techniques, EEG comes to mind first because simple mobile devices with a limited number of electrodes are already commercially available. If, by combining fMRI and EEG in the laboratory, we can detect EEG signatures that reflect the modulation of the targeted brain networks by our patients during neurofeedback, we could then train them to influence these EEG parameters directly and continue with these exercises in their homes. This will probably work best for superficial parts of the brain whose activity can be picked up easily by EEG. For example, once patients with PD have successfully learnt to up-regulate their SMA through fMRI-NF, they may also be able to modulate their sensorimotor rhythm in the EEG to achieve similar clinical benefits. Combination with EEG is less straightforward for areas deep in the brain, such as the basal ganglia, because signals from these areas lose strength and are distorted when travelling through the brain to be picked up by EEG electrodes on the scalp.

For mental and behavioural disorders, in particular, an innovative way of delivering feedback may be through the smartphone. Although a smartphone will not directly record brain activity (although it could potentially pick up signals from a wireless EEG cap through a Bluetooth connection) it can deliver nudges that are related to the neurofeedback protocol. For example, if patients with depression report that imagining calming landscape scenes is an effective way of up-regulating networks associated with positive emotions, such pictures can be delivered on the smartphone during daily training sessions.

Smartphones can be programmed to create closed loops of behaviour control. Through their inbuilt sensors (for example, an accelerometer) and functionalities (for example, GPS location services) they can track an individual's movements, whereabouts, daily activity patterns and social interactions. Researchers in the School of Computer Science at Cardiff University, led by Roger Whitaker, are combining this information with personality tests to create profiles of social behaviour (Figure 3.5). The information collected by the smartphone could also be used to identify triggers and antecedents of dysfunctional behaviour, for example drinking relapses or binge eating, or stressful situations, for example anxiety-provoking scenarios. Once the smartphone (or the algorithms governing its function) has been trained to detect these situations based on its multi-channel signals, it can also be programmed to send the appropriate nudges for behaviour change or remind the patient to engage in coping strategies, for example relaxing visual imagery learnt during neurofeedback.

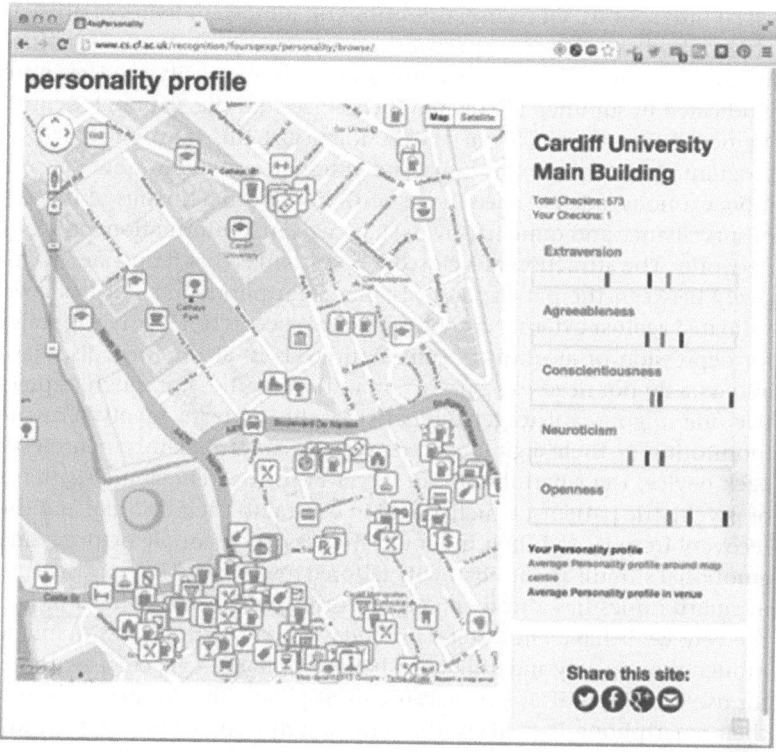

Figure 3.5 The Foursquare personality experiment hosted at Cardiff University collects personality profiles from users of the mobile social network Foursquare

Note: Users rate themselves along the standard personality dimensions of extraversion, agreeableness, conscientiousness, neuroticism and openness. This allows possible correlations between movement activity and personality type to be discovered, along with providing a base for extrapolating a sense of the 'personality' of individual venues. For example, this user seems to be more extraverted than the average visitor to the University Main Building; conversely the average visitor to Cardiff City Centre, which is famous for its bars and clubs, is even more extraverted. Figure courtesy of Professor Roger Whitaker, Cardiff University. For further information see: http://www.cs.cf.ac.uk/recognition/foursqexp.

The smartphone, whose use has become pervasive over the last few years (in 2013 the majority of mobile phones in the UK were smartphones), offers unique potential for the monitoring of activities in everyday settings. This includes basic activities that are highly relevant to mental health, such as sleeping, eating and drinking, and complex social interactions. Of course, this brings up important issues of privacy. Those who have always suspected that our physical and social activities are being monitored via our smartphones by the security services, were vindicated in summer 2013 when it emerged that the National Security Agency (NSA) of the USA had been doing just this through its PRISM program. Although smartphone and internet users may now become more cautious, most of them have, until now, been oblivious to the risk of surveillance and quite happy to share personal information via social networks. The attraction of a closed loop system is that it operates exclusively between the patient and his/ her smartphone, once it has been validated against external criteria of clinical success (such as rating scales for depression or alcohol consumption levels in alcohol use disorder), and data do not need to be passed on to third parties (although in practice one might want to get the patient's clinical team involved in the monitoring of their digital experiences). As an ambulatory neurofeedback device, the smartphone can target both the behavioural patterns of psychiatric patients, which are often central to their disorder and the recovery from it, and their inner experiences, for example by providing emotional stimuli and individually tailored memories. The pervasive use of smartphones has already changed norms of accepted behaviour and the way we behave and interact in a day-to-day setting. This dramatic influence on society and individual behaviour has not yet been exploited for use in mental disorders. Because most people like to spend time on their smartphone it is likely that any smartphone-based intervention will attain good compliance. It is therefore surprising that the use of the smartphone in mental health (and healthcare in general) has lagged far behind its use in general society. It is likely that this gap will be filled soon, if only because of the huge commercial potential in developing specific applications for a market of hundreds of millions of people who are affected by a mental illness.

4
The Ethics and Politics of Brain Control

4.1 Brain control in neurology and psychiatry

The two largest programmes (in terms of the number of treated patients) of invasive brain control were the lobotomies of the 1940s and 1950s and the DBS treatment of Parkinson's disease that started in the early 1990s. Both included over 50,000 patients, and the number of PD patients receiving DBS is continuously increasing. However, their standing in public and scientific perception could not be more different. To most commentators, lobotomy epitomises all that is or was bad about psychiatry, including crude and non-scientific disease models and procedures, authoritarian doctors and coercive procedures in mental institutions. Conversely, DBS is considered to be a modern procedure, based on quantifiable physiological disease models. It epitomises the future of medicine, in which the most recent advances in computer technology and bioengineering are harnessed to push the boundaries of new therapies.

Surgical approaches to schizophrenia were abandoned several decades ago. Then amongst the most controversial procedures in the second wave of psychiatric surgery in the 1960s and 1970s, amygdalotomies are now performed very rarely[147] and hypothalamotomies seem to have disappeared completely. Psychiatric surgery has survived through the stereotactic procedures that were developed in the wake of the open leucotomies, mainly cingulotomy and anterior capsulotomy for patients with obsessive compulsive disorder (OCD) and depression who do not respond to standard treatments. These procedures are still performed in several specialised centres worldwide, for example Massachusetts General Hospital in the USA, Dundee University in Scotland and Yonsei University in Seoul, South Korea. Outside this orthodox psychiatric surgery for OCD and depression, several groups have expanded the indication of these procedures to include behavioural disorders, mainly addiction. The large cingulotomy programme active in St Petersburg, Russia, from 1999 to 2003 is probably the most striking example of this development, but we have also encountered programmes of destructive surgery of the nucleus accumbens for heroin addiction in Chinese hospitals (Section 2.11).

DBS for movement disorders is now firmly established in clinical practice, although access varies widely across the world. Because recent trial data already suggest benefits in early PD it is likely that the number of patients considered for DBS will increase further in countries where DBS is available. There is already a big divide in the management of PD between countries with highly developed health systems and those, for example in most of Sub-Saharan Africa, where the majority of patients are still undiagnosed and untreated. Yet increasing life expectancy in the economically developing parts of the world implies that they will face an increasing challenge from neurodegenerative diseases.[148] For these countries, the focus in the foreseeable future is likely to be on widening access to diagnosis and treatment with medication and low-technology rehabilitation, such as exercise groups, rather than on the development of DBS programmes. Conversely, countries with established DBS programmes will have to decide whether to make the procedure more widely available to patients in earlier stages of the disease. It has to be remembered, though, that the rates of surgical side effects, such as bleeds and infections, are still considerable and can affect up to 20% of patients.[149] The British National Institute for Clinical Excellence (NICE), which advises the National Health Service on the cost effectiveness of therapies, has estimated that up to 10% of PD patients are suitable for surgery. If, in a very crude estimate, the results of the EARLYSTIM trial discussed in Section 2.5 were to double this figure to 20%, this would mean that approximately 6,000 additional patients could be considered, at a cost of £180 million (and entailing the need to train many more surgeons in functional neurosurgery). In economic terms, this might be offset by reductions in other treatment costs and higher productivity and longer lives of the patients. However, it is likely that any commissioning bodies will demand evidence from more trials, including a longer follow-up in these early PD groups and a formal assessment of economic impacts, before recommending a wider rollout of DBS. It is also worth remembering that the purpose of using DBS in early as opposed to advanced PD is somewhat different. In advanced PD, the main purpose is the reduction of dyskinesias and major motor disability,[150] whereas in early PD, where normally these problems have not yet become manifest, the main purpose is the reduction of dopaminergic medication (without loss of motor function or, ideally, with even better function than on the pre-operative dose). What is largely unknown is whether other, non-invasive neuromodulatory approaches could potentially have a similar benefit. It is certainly worth exploring whether the modulation of brain plasticity with non-invasive electromagnetic stimulation (Transcranial Magnetic or Electrical Stimulation, TMS or TES) in conjunction with exercise can enable patients to reduce their daily medication. Neurofeedback is another possible avenue that might lead to a reduced need for medication. If patients can be trained to recruit compensatory circuits for movement initiation and control they could potentially attain a similar level of motor function in the on state with a reduced dose of dopaminergic medication. Furthermore, the combination of physical (exercise), physiological (brain self-regulation) and psychological (mental imagery and simulation) strategies that are trained during neurofeedback might even give them better motor control in the off state (for an explanation of "on" and "off" periods see Section 2.4). One might envisage a scenario where patients first go through a course of non-invasive neuromodulation, for example neurofeedback, for three to six months with the expectation that some of them will experience a relevant gain of motor function and quality of living (and potentially an accompanying reduction in dopaminergic medication). Invasive procedures such as DBS would then only be considered for patients who do not benefit from a self-regulation regime. Even if this necessitated the purchase of an equivalent of ten new MR scanners (assuming 2,500 scan hours per year and five sessions of neurofeedback per person, one scanner can support interventions for 500 patients per year), at £15 million this would still be an order of magnitude cheaper than a DBS programme for early PD, and it would be cost effective if it made implantation superfluous in just one in ten DBS candidates. However, healthcare funders will want to see very good clinical evidence for improvements in motor function and quality of life after neurofeedback before considering such an investment.

Compared to DBS for movement disorders, psychiatric DBS is still a rather small field. Around 100 patients each have been treated in published studies of DBS for OCD and depression, and the numbers for other potential psychiatric indications are even lower. Psychiatric DBS has mainly been applied to those mental disorders which had, at some point, been approached with destructive surgery. The anatomical targets were chosen on the basis of four sources of evidence:

- Targets where clinical benefits had been observed after destructive surgery, for example the internal capsule in OCD.
- Targets where clinical benefits had been observed after DBS for neurological disorders, for example the subthalamic nucleus in OCD.
- Targets where abnormal activation had been postulated on the basis of functional imaging studies, for example the subgenual cingulate gyrus in depression.
- Targets that were identified largely in animal models, for example the nucleus accumbens as a potential target for DBS in addiction.

It is not clear at the moment which of these approaches is clinically most promising. Several further trials of DBS for OCD and depression are under way, and most activity in this area has happened in the USA, France, Germany and the Netherlands. If these trials produce consistent outcome data that are at least as good as those from cingulotomy and capsulotomy studies it is likely that destructive surgery for OCD and depression will be gradually abandoned in favour of DBS because of its presumed reversibility and better public image (on which more to follow).

Depression is unique in the group of diseases treated with DBS in that it typically has a relapsing-remitting course. The other diseases are generally either chronic or progressive. For example, one would not expect any real improvement in untreated severe OCD, and patients with untreated PD invariably experience a decline in their motor functions. Conversely, patients with depression generally get better after some time, even without treatment. Although patients who are considered for DBS or surgery normally have a longstanding diagnosis of depression and do not respond to any other treatment they can still get better spontaneously. The confounding effect of spontaneous recovery is a problem for any evaluation of treatment effects in depression. The normal way of dealing with this problem in clinical trials is to include groups of patients who receive treatment as usual or a placebo treatment, because these patients should show the same rate of spontaneous remission as the patients receiving the active treatment. So far, this has not been standard in DBS trials for depression, and reasonably large groups of patients would be needed to make such a comparison meaningful. An alternative would be to provide evidence for specific treatment effects through immediate clinical improvements occurring during the initial stimulation. Dramatic improvements in motor function directly at stimulation onset can be observed in PD and dystonia, but nothing of this sort has so far been reported for DBS in depression. Stimulation of the subgenual cingulate has led to immediate effects of higher alertness and motivation in some cases,[111] and stimulation of the medial forebrain bundle in a recent German study[114] elicited immediate "appetitive orienting" in some patients, which can be interpreted as heightened motivation, although mood still took several weeks to improve. To be fair to the proponents of DBS, the delay in its action is actually not all that different from widely used antidepressant drugs, which also take several weeks to improve mood.

It is perhaps surprising that the hypothalamic regions where stimulation (and self-stimulation) elicited such pleasurable effects in Heath's patients (see Section 2.3) have not been targeted with DBS for depression, but perhaps today's neurosurgeons are wary of these effects because they had not been replicated in later cases of hypothalamic stimulation for other indications. Furthermore, Heath's studies were generally focused on short-term effects. Making long-term DBS dependent on immediate hedonic responses would create the risk of dependence. People, like rats, have a tendency to want more of the stuff they like. If DBS induces immediate feelings of pleasure patients may demand more. If we use the analogy of substance dependence, this might entail the need to ramp up stimulation intensities over time to maintain the hedonic effect. Obviously, increasing the current that flows through the DBS electrode increases the risk of damage to the stimulated part of the brain and also the chance of creating undesirable effects by stimulating neighbouring areas. Avoiding tolerance in DBS programmes is therefore paramount. As yet, modern DBS studies have not reported such a need to increase the intensity of stimulation (unlike in historic self-stimulation studies, where patients increased stimulation frequency to hedonic areas when given the opportunity).

Almost all the clinical domains of former or current psychiatric surgery have now come within the reach of DBS programmes. DBS of the nucleus accumbens for addiction is currently being tested in three trials (two for opiate and one for alcohol addiction) in Germany and China, DBS for obesity in one trial at Ohio State University in the USA, and DBS for anorexia nervosa in two trials in Canada and China, according to the online database for clinical trials, clinicaltrials.gov, accessed on 22 July 2013. There is even one pilot trial targeting the negative symptoms of schizophrenia with DBS of the nucleus accumbens or VTA, run from the University of Toronto, Canada. A new indication for DBS would be PTSD, where, based on animal models, two targets have been proposed, the amygdala[151] and the bed nucleus of the stria terminalis (BNST),[152] which is a relay station between the amygdala, ventral tegmentum and hypothalamus. Conversely, at present no programme seems to be investigating the potential effects of DBS of the hypothalamus on paedophilia, which is perhaps not surprising considering the high amount of controversy the relevant surgical programme had generated in the 1960s and 1970s.

However, a recent report from Spain on six patients who underwent bilateral DBS of the hypothalamus (its posteromedial part) for pathological aggression[153] shows that Sano's sedative neurosurgery programme of the 1960s (see Section 2.9) is now being continued with brain stimulation technology. The group in Madrid operated on adult patients with severe developmental delay and learning disability who were aggressive towards others and themselves. Some, but not all, of these patients also had epilepsy. Because of the low intelligence of the patients the surgeons obtained consent from their parents or legal guardians. They reported behavioural improvement, for example in aggression levels and self-injuring behaviour, in five of the six patients. Some of the patients also became more manageable and could be discharged from their residential institutions into family care over weekends. Yet, expectedly there was no improvement in patient IQ, and patients did remain heavily reliant on care. Moreover, two of the patients died (reportedly of causes unrelated to the DBS) before follow-up could be completed. A similar procedure was used by Italian neurosurgeons Angelo Franzini and Giovanni Broggi for aggressive behaviour in severely intellectually impaired patients. The IQ of the six patients whose outcomes they reported in 2009 was 40 or below or not measurable. An IQ below 40 equates to a severe learning disability. Some of the patients operated on by Franzini and Broggi had been impaired from birth, whereas others had suffered from brain damage in later life after injury or cardiac arrest. Bilateral DBS of the posteromedial hypothalamus reduced levels of aggressive behaviour, and some of the patients could be discharged from hospital into therapeutic communities or re-integrated into their families. The surgeons also reported that the frequency of epileptic seizures decreased in the two patients who were also suffering from epilepsy.[154] Thus, surgical control of behaviour in patients who are unable to consent for themselves remains a relevant issue in current ethical debates.

4.2 The ethics of psychiatric surgery

Although its scale is now much reduced compared to the heyday of lobotomy in the 1940s and 1950s psychiatric surgery in its modern, more targeted and circumscribed form, is a reality of contemporary medicine. Whereas the cingulotomy and capsulotomy programmes for OCD and depression in the USA and UK now only include small numbers of patients, surgery for addiction seems to be on the rise, particularly in China, and an ever expanding range of indications is being proposed for DBS. Yet many people have concerns about operative interventions for psychiatric disorders. It is somewhat surprising that we are not seeing a repetition of the heated ethical and political debates of the 1970s and the most likely explanation is that the revival of psychosurgery has remained largely unnoticed by the general public.

Psychiatric surgery is tarnished by the history of lobotomy. Lobotomy is now widely regarded as an inhumane programme with little scientific foundation that coerced patients into mutilating operations and left them apathetic and cognitively impaired, for the sake of making it easier to manage underfunded psychiatric hospitals. Although this view is exaggerated – because these programmes were initiated largely because of a lack of other treatment options in the pre-pharmacological era of psychiatry, and some of the outcome data initially looked promising – the experience of lobotomy still brings up ethical issues that are relevant today. These include the questions of consent, scientific foundation, irreversibility, risk/benefit ratios and risk of misuse. How we assess the benefits and risks worth taking is a difficult and highly culture-dependent issue in its own right. Just looking at one example of an evaluation of lobotomy shows how attitudes have shifted in this respect. Sargant and Slater tersely summarised an American study from 1943 as having a particularly good risk/benefit ratio: "of 582 patients, mostly schizophrenia, treated in the U.S.A., there were only 11 deaths from the operation while 235 were got back to work."[155] Today we would be concerned about a procedure with approximately 2% mortality if its main justification was put in socioeconomic terms. Of course, it is possible that a patient may be prepared to accept this 2% risk when faced with an operation that has a reasonable chance of helping him or her get out of the grip of a debilitating mental illness and allowing him or her to re-integrate in society. One of the main shifts of attitude over the last 60 years has been that clinicians are neither prepared for, nor in a position to make such decisions on behalf of their patients, and that patient choice has become a paramount principle in psychiatric treatments.

Who can consent to psychiatric surgery?

One of the fundamental standards of medical ethics today is that any treatment needs the consent of the patient. The only exceptions apply in cases where the patient cannot be consulted about emergency treatment, for example when he or she is in coma, or in cases where the patient lacks insight into the medical necessity of a treatment because of mental disorder or cognitive impairment and the doctor consults advocates acting on their behalf, or a court of law.

Because of the radical nature of surgical intervention for psychiatric disorders and the particular concerns about potential coercion of mentally ill (and thus more vulnerable) patients, the procedures for obtaining consent and additional safeguards are now even stricter than those applied in general medicine. The National Commission for the Protection of Human Subjects of Biomedical and Behavioral Research in the USA, which drew up the first general guidelines for psychiatric surgery in 1977, recommended that such procedures should only be performed at institutions with an Institutional Review Board (IRB) approved by the Department of Health. The duties of the IRB were to check that the procedure was appropriate to the individual case, that the patient had given consent and that adequate pre- and post-operative evaluations would be performed. Bioethicist George Annas thought that these safeguards did not go far enough because the IRB could determine capacity to consent by hearsay, without actually interviewing the patient in person.[156] The National Commission ruled out any psychiatric surgery against the objection of the patient but also recommended specific additional safeguards for patients that it regarded as particularly vulnerable to coercion: children, prisoners, patients who were detained in mental hospitals against their will, patients with a legal guardian, and those incapable of giving consent themselves. These safeguards involved setting up a National Psychosurgery Advisory Board that would determine whether the operation had benefits for the psychiatric symptoms or disorder of the patient. In addition, the patient or his/her guardian (or parent in the case of children) had to consent to the procedure, and it had to be approved by a court. Finally, for inpatients or prison inmates, the operation should be performed in a hospital separate from the institution where the patient was confined. However, other commentators of the time (e.g. O'Callaghan and Carroll, see Section 2.9[85]) wanted to rule out psychiatric surgery on prison inmates altogether because they felt that coercion could never be ruled out in this context.

Interestingly, it does not appear that such a National Advisory Board, which would be convened upon the application of the surgeon wanting to operate on patients from the most vulnerable groups, was ever established in the USA. Other jurisdictions, for example Australia and India,[157] have established such National Boards for general scrutiny of psychiatric surgery programmes. The report of one such board, the Psychosurgery Review Board of the Australian State of Victoria shows an interesting trend. Having received no applications in 2001–2006, the Board received, on average, two applications per year in 2007–2012 owing to the rise of DBS (www.mhrb.vic.gov.au, accessed on 29 September 2013).

Unlike programmes in the 1960s and 1970s, current psychiatric surgery (including DBS) programmes do not seem to include children, involuntary patients or prisoners, at least according to the published reports, but DBS has been performed on patients unable to consent for themselves. The recent study of hypothalamic DBS for aggressive behaviour from Spain, which relied on consent from parents or guardians, cited the following criteria "to ensure patient protection":

> involvement of an experienced multidisciplinary team, careful selection of severely afflicted patients with conditions that are refractory to other treatment, careful explanation of the purpose and risks of the procedures to parents and legal guardians, and approval from an institutional review board or a local ethics committee that oversees the observance of national and international regulations.[153]

Although the Madrid group thus implemented the majority of the criteria of the American commission, they did not incorporate the additional safeguards of review by a National Advisory Board and approval by a court. Because the number of patients in recent studies of surgery for behaviour control has been small and any outcome data are therefore preliminary it would seem prudent to coordinate these types of studies at national level (or at the level of international bodies such as the European Union or World Health Organisation, WHO). Furthermore, in light of the high rate of deaths in the Spanish study (two out of six patients), although they were reportedly unrelated to the intervention, it would seem reasonable to require scrutiny of individual cases by a court of law to protect both the patients and their clinicians.

The scientific foundation for cutting "healthy tissue"

Valenstein criticised German hypothalamotomies in sexual offenders based on the argument that there was insufficient evidence for the existence of a sex centre, let alone separate male and female sex centres in the human hypothalamus. O'Callaghan and Carroll's verdict on the theoretical basis of most psychosurgical procedures was similarly damning: "Psychosurgeons have tended to resort to rather loose and tenuous allegories as a substitute for direct and sophisticated physiological theory." They lamented that most psychiatric surgeons subscribed to an outdated model of strict functional localisation, targeting specific brain structures to modify specific behaviours when "the behavioural targets of psychosurgery are complex psychological processes, maintained by intricate arrangements of events in the environment and serviced by a system of cerebral structures working in a concerted and dynamic fashion". Today we would call this a network model. Based on this model of interconnectedness of functional circuits in the brain, they concluded that "it would seem unreasonable to suppose that psychosurgery can ever aspire to specific effects".[85] This view was actually implicit in the approach of American neurosurgeon William Scoville, who stated in 1972 that "there is no need to vary the location of operation for neuroses, depressions, schizophrenia, or psychic pain."[158] From today's perspective, there is some justification in Scoville's claim because lesions in the same area (or DBS) can have effects on very different disorders. The reported success of operations targeting the ventral striatum for OCD, depression and opiate dependence is just one particularly striking example. Of course, areas like the ventral striatum may be crucial for a variety of disease processes, but this success may also rely on non-specific effects of the stimulation or even on placebo effects. Another example of this philosophy is the recent attempt to use DBS of the subgenual cingulate in patients with anorexia. In the original DBS studies of depression the subgenual cingulate was chosen as the target because some imaging results had indicated metabolic changes in this region in patients who recovered from depression. No such neurobiological foundation was available for targeting this area in anorexia. Perhaps this difference explains why DBS of the subgenual cingulate has led to clinical responses – at least initially – in over 50% of patients, whereas improvement in anorexia has been much less impressive. After all, not all psychiatric disorders are created equal with regard to their brain substrates. The problem is that for most psychiatric disorders we still know very little about the affected brain areas and the underlying physiological mechanisms.

Although some of the more recent psychiatric surgery programmes have tried to build up a foundation of imaging studies to pinpoint potentially dysfunctional nodes in the network of contributing areas, it is as true as it was in the days of lobotomy that the operations are not based on any direct evidence that the targeted area is diseased. The procedures to identify potential targets for surgery have become more sophisticated than in the days of Fulton and Moniz, when observations of altered behaviour in one or two monkeys were deemed to be a sufficient basis for a large-scale intervention programme in humans. However, when we use neuroimaging techniques, such as positron emission tomography or fMRI, to identify hotspots of altered activation in patients with depression or OCD this still does not allow us to identify pathological areas in individual cases. The critique that psychiatric surgeons are cutting healthy tissue (or at least tissue which they have no way of proving is affected by the disease) therefore still applies. This constitutes an important difference from epilepsy surgery, which generally relies on the demonstration of abnormal structures and/or functions in the targeted area of the individual patient's brain. Thus, psychiatric surgeons still largely operate in *terra incognita*.

This "blind" approach does not necessarily make psychiatric surgery unethical. The widespread practice of prescribing psychotropic drugs to people with mental illness is similarly blind. For example, over 50 million people worldwide are prescribed antidepressants from the class of selective serotonin reuptake inhibitors (SSRI). These drugs increase the availability of the neurotransmitter serotonin in the synaptic cleft, the space between nerve cells. Although it has been known for 60 years that drugs acting on the serotonin system can alleviate depression we still have no good model that explains why this is the case. The most straightforward explanation – that patients with depression have a deficit in serotonin – can probably be ruled out. SSRIs, not unlike psychiatric surgery, therefore constitute a treatment for depression that works in a reasonable number of cases, although its mechanism of action is shrouded in mystery. This does not only apply to drug treatment and surgery since the scientific basis for all other treatments in psychiatry, for example electroconvulsive therapy (ECT) or various types of psychotherapy, is similarly sketchy.

Althoug other treatments, particularly ECT and drugs, have received their fair share of criticism psychiatric surgery has been attacked particularly heavily. There is a deep seated, and justifiable, reservation about invasive and irreversible procedures, and medicine generally requires a particularly high level of evidence before they are sanctioned. For example, in an emergency setting one might administer two antibiotic drugs to a patient with a life-threatening infection arising from a gangrenous foot, knowing that only one of them will be effective, rather than wait several hours until the germ responsible for the infection has been identified. But one would not easily amputate both feet before having determined which one is actually affected.

Are psychiatric diseases curable?

One of the fundamental distinctions of medical therapies is that between curative and palliative procedures. This distinction is most familiar from the field of cancer where a curative treatment is intended to remove all cancerous tissue – through surgery, drugs and/or radiation – and thus cure the patient completely of the cancer. Conversely, palliative procedures are intended to alleviate the discomfort associated with the cancer, for example by removing a tumour that is causing pain, without the aim of curing the patient of the cancer completely. Palliative procedures are considered when the curative approach would involve a very high surgical risk or when it just would not be possible to remove all cancerous tissue. Palliative procedures are intended to make the patient's remaining months or years more comfortable and less painful. In other words, they put a cloak (Latin: *pallium*) around the disease to shield the patient from its most dire consequences.

O'Callaghan and Carroll introduced this curative/palliative distinction into the psychosurgery debate. They classified psychiatric surgery as an "essentially palliative measure" because even the modern, stereotactic approaches would at best produce "non-specific, generalized outcomes".[85] The analogy with cancer would be that an operation would not remove the source of the symptoms, it would just produce behavioural effects (such as placidity) to make them more bearable for the patient and those around him or her. Some of the descriptions of the effects of leucotomy indeed referred to predominantly palliative effects:

> Unless mutilating operations are performed, leucotomy has only three main effects: tension is reduced, the patient becomes less concerned with his symptoms, and he cannot keep his mind fixed for so long on any particular train of thought or action. ... Delusions may die out for lack of emotional reinforcement, or, if maintained, are held with lesser force and concern. Hallucinations very often persist, but worry the patient less.[155]

O'Callaghan & Carroll considered the palliative/ curative distinction as being relevant to the ethical evaluation: "while risky curative procedures are ethically permissible, risky palliative procedures are not". Although this general statement is reasonable the classification of psychiatric surgery as "palliative" is probably not entirely fair. In psychiatry, unlike cancer, we have no measurable physical indicators of treatment success, such as the reduction of tumour size or the decrease of a particular biomarker, but the symptoms and their behavioural and functional consequences are all that matters for the assessment of treatment outcome. A non-specific outcome that helped patients across a range of mental disorders cope better with their problems and stressors could thus be very helpful and, indeed, almost "curative". In fact, many psychotherapeutic approaches have just this aim, and even successful drug treatment may not necessarily address the root causes of the symptoms. Many patients report that antipsychotic drugs help them cope better with some of their symptoms, or that antidepressants "take the edge off" their worries and anxieties. Admittedly, the risk of life-threatening adverse effects is higher with psychiatric surgery (including DBS) than with psychiatric drugs, let alone psychotherapy. One would thus demand that surgical procedures show a higher effectiveness than other approaches (or effectiveness in treatment-refractory patients). Yet, if a surgical treatment for depression or schizophrenia could indeed lead to a considerable reduction in disease burden and suicide risk, and improve health, behaviour and social functioning, it could become one of the most "curative" procedures available to psychiatry. The likely gain in life expectancy from such a treatment could then be weighed up against the mortality risk from surgery, similar to the practice in other areas of surgery for chronic disease, such as cancer or ischaemic heart disease. Bypass surgery is certainly not curative in the sense that it restores a patient's coronary vessels to their original pristine state, but it entails a reasonable workaround that increases life expectancy with a good quality of life for many patients, and nobody would call it palliative. If someone developed a psychiatric equivalent of bypass surgery, patients with severe and sometimes life-threatening mental disorders, such as depression, OCD, schizophrenia or anorexia, who have not responded to less risky treatments, should not be denied it just because it cannot be shown to attack the root cause of their symptoms. These considerations show that, ultimately, the main factor when considering the ethics of psychiatric surgery is its effectiveness rather than its theoretical basis.

How can we find out whether psychiatric surgery works?

The question of whether the large lobotomy programmes of the 1940s and 1950s were effective is now mainly of historical interest, and has little practical consequence because no neurosurgeon nowadays would consider open lobotomy or leucotomy for any psychiatric disorder. As pointed out in Section 2.9, the question of the effectiveness of lobotomy is also very difficult to answer. Although very large follow-up studies were conducted, and often reported positive outcomes, these generally relied on the subjective impressions of the treating physicians and included no comparison with control groups. Even if we accepted the evidence from these studies it would have relatively little bearing on present-day clinical decision-making because psychiatric surgery is now considered only for patients who do not respond to the standard drug treatments, which were not available in the lobotomy era. In fact, even the most optimistic psychiatric commentators on leucotomy acknowledged that it was not particularly effective in schizophrenia patients who came to surgery several years after disease onset and after affective flattening and other prominent negative symptoms had set in.[155] Today's refractory schizophrenia patients would therefore be unlikely to respond to destructive surgery even if it was available.

The evaluation of stereotactic procedures is more relevant for today's psychiatrists when considering surgery for their patients. Most studies of cingulotomy and capsulotomy for OCD or depression have reported sustained response rates around 50%, although without control groups we cannot rule out placebo effects and we do not know what proportion of patients would have recovered spontaneously. In their 1982 survey O'Callaghan and Carroll concluded that "only obsessional neurosis and sexual deviation would seem to attract high reported percentage improvement rates" (but urged caution in relation to the latter because only just over 30 cases had been formally reported and some of the assessments had been questionable in their view).[85]

Although the mortality (death rate) associated with modern psychiatric surgery appears to be relatively low (under 1%), non-lethal complications, such as intracranial bleeds, infections (particularly problematic in DBS procedures, where by the very nature of the procedure foreign material is left in the brain) and postoperative epilepsy need to be taken into account. The occasional reports of suicide after psychiatric surgery and DBS (including DBS for non-psychiatric indications) are also of some concern. Although the numbers of patients affected (only one or two per study at most) were too small to allow for definitive conclusions as to whether suicides occur more frequently after cingulotomy or DBS than in patients with the respective disorders who are not treated in this way, it will certainly be important to inform patients of this risk and embed any intervention in a programme of careful postoperative psychiatric monitoring. One particular concern with invasive interventions for severe mental illness, in which patients will necessarily invest a great amount of hope, is the despair and frustration that can arise if the procedure does not have the desired effect. This outcome could considerably worsen a pre-existing mood disorder and constitute a suicide risk in its own right.[159]

If we apply the same ethical criteria to psychiatric surgery as to any other branch of medicine – informed consent, careful assessment of the risk/benefit ratio, pre- and postoperative monitoring and ongoing evaluation – there is no reason for a wholesale ban on this type of procedure. The recommendations of the American National Commission of 1977 still provide useful guidance. Because psychiatric surgery (including DBS) is still experimental (meaning that its effects have not been supported by definitive controlled trials) it should only be performed in specialist academic centres with appropriate long-term monitoring and scientific evaluation. Because of the invasive and irreversible nature of the procedure special care needs to be taken to assess a patient's ability to provide free and informed consent, for example through the committees established under the Mental Health Act in England and Wales (see Section 2.10). Although the National Commission of the USA only recommended a National Advisory Board for the protection of specific groups of patients, it would be preferable to establish such boards generally to provide advice on psychiatric surgery (and DBS). Such boards could also collect information on the less well-established surgical procedures and indications, for example the destruction of the nucleus accumbens in patients with opiate addiction practiced in China, and make specific recommendations. They could also oversee the prospective trials that are needed to gain more information about the effectiveness of the different surgical approaches. Another very useful recommendation of the National Commission was "that a mechanism be set up on the national level to collect data on psychosurgery". This could also cover the expanding practice of psychiatric DBS and collect data on clinical outcome, adverse effects and subjective patient experience. Such a "neuromodulation experience registry" would provide a more balanced view of the actual effects in practice than would published trial reports, which tend to be biased in favour of positive outcomes.[160]

Some commentators have rejected the need for controlled trials of psychiatric surgery,[85] for two opposing reasons. One of these extreme positions is that the evidence for the effectiveness of psychiatric surgery is already so strong that trials would be redundant; at the other extreme, it has been argued that its theoretical basis is so poor that it would be irresponsible to operate on any further patients. However, the mainstream position is that trials are needed because the clinical problems addressed

by psychiatric surgery are still pressing and some of the reports in literature have been promising, but often lacked the rigour of formal trials.
One particularly interesting way of conducting such trials would be to
compare destructive surgery with DBS, because most of the expected
placebo effects (from an invasive procedure, detailed follow-up and
attention from medical teams) would be similar, ideally with a matched,
treatment as usual group as a comparator for spontaneous remission. It
would also be of interest to compare surgical approaches with a control
intervention that involves the same amount of individual attention
and use of high-tech machinery, for example Transcranial Magnetic
Stimulation.

Surgery for "behavioural disorders"

Surgery to control abnormal – addictive, aggressive or sexually deviant –
behaviour is particularly controversial. The largest body of clinical
experience is available for aggressive and auto-aggressive (self-injuring)
behaviour. Although current programmes (such as the Madrid study of
hypothalamic DBS mentioned above) are confined to adult patients,
surgeons in the 1960s and 1970s operated on children with severe behavioural disorders, regardless of whether they were affected by epilepsy
or not. An Austrian group at Graz University applied lesions to the
amygdala on one side and the dorsomedial nucleus of the thalamus on
the other. They operated on six children, aged 8–17, who were suffering
from severe developmental delay, with severe self-injurious behaviour
that could not be controlled by medication. Half of the patients also
had evidence of epileptic activity on the EEG. In three of their patients
they observed a reduction in auto-aggressive behaviour, which made it
possible to reduce their medication. The authors reported that in some
cases even the straitjackets that the young patients previously had to wear
could be removed.[161] This case series exemplifies the main ethical issues
in the psychosurgery debate: whether it should be applied to children;
whether operations should be conducted without evidence of an organic
pathology; and how to ensure that surgery really benefits the patients
rather than serves the interests of those who have to manage them in
hospitals or care homes. It is interesting to note the different attitudes of
the medical community to these matters, which today would doubtless
feature very strongly in any debate on surgery for behaviour management. However, when the Austrian doctors presented their study at the
Second International Symposium on Stereoencephalotomy in Vienna
in 1965, the ensuing discussion brought up many technical details of
the optimal and safest surgical procedure, but did not even touch on

issues of consent and appropriateness of the indication. A recent paper summarised the issue from a neurosurgical perspective:

> Advances in neuropharmacology during the last 3 decades, along with the skepticism regarding the surgical treatment of psychiatric disorders, have led to the abandonment of stereotactic amygdalotomy in treating patients with severe aggression or self-mutilation disorders. Note, however, that certain cases of violent behavioral disorders that do not respond to any other treatment modality might benefit from stereotactic amygdalotomy. Medically refractory cases of aggressive, assaultive behavior or of self-mutilation resistant to appropriate pharmacological or behavioural treatment may improve with stereotactic amygdalotomy. The introduction of high-field MR imaging units in routine clinical practice, in which the amygdaloid nuclei can be nicely identified, and the development of frameless neuronavigational systems of high accuracy can make stereotactic amygdalotomy an appealing treatment option in these patients. A team of experienced psychiatrists and a functional neurosurgeon very familiar with psychosurgical procedures should select appropriate surgical candidates. It cannot be overemphasized that this procedure should be considered only in extreme cases after exhausting all other therapeutic options and only when the patient and his or her family are fully aware of the potential outcome and risks of the procedure.[162]

Although all these points are reasonable the problem is that we are concerned here with patients who mostly do not have the intellectual capacity to understand the impact of such an operation and therefore would not be able to consent for themselves. These patients are particularly vulnerable because of their severe learning disabilities and because they are mostly institutionalised. Another ethical problem is that the success of such an operation would generally be measured by the responses of family and professional carers, rather than the patient's self-assessment of their well-being. Because most of the patients in question are severely impaired in their communication abilities, the impact of the surgery on their feelings is judged from their observed behaviour, for example, diminished frequency of self-harming. In sum, these patients are subjected to an operation that interferes with outwardly healthy brain tissue, to which they lack the capacity to consent and whose outcome they often cannot be asked to assess. In this scenario, the additional safeguards of approval of the general procedure by a specialist National Advisory Board and approval of individual cases by a court of law are crucial.

The main argument against surgical intervention to treat sexual offenders was also based on issues of consent. Although the hypothalamotomies of the 1960s and 1970s showed promising results in some reports (see Section 2.9) this programme came to a halt in Germany in the 1970s chiefly because of concerns about the freedom of the consent obtained from patients who were detained or faced with legal proceedings because of sexual offences. Another concern, perhaps more specific to the cultural climate of the 1970s, was that the surgeons were trying to cure abnormal behaviour with a brain intervention rather than with behavioural or other psychological techniques. Today there is probably a greater willingness within the clinical professions to accept that brain and behaviour are inextricably linked and that the distinction between behavioural, mental and brain disorders is often not clear cut. It is therefore surprising that disorders of sexual behaviour are not amongst the disorders considered for psychiatric surgery today.

Surgery for sexual aggression came very close to a formal trial, which would have been one of the most rigorous tests ever conducted of psychiatric surgery because it involved a control group undergoing a standard therapy. In 1972 two doctors at the Lafayette Clinic in Detroit, Ernest Rodin and Jacques Gottlieb, obtained funding from the state of Michigan to conduct a comparison of amygalotomy and anti-androgen treatment in 24 sexual offenders from the State's mental health system. However, it proved difficult to recruit patients, partly because a statute allowing for the detention of "Criminal Sexual Psychopaths" had recently been repealed and many potential candidates had been released from the institutions. Thus, the doctors were left with only one potential patient, a 35-year old known only as John Doe during the subsequent legal proceedings. John Doe had been charged in 1955 with the rape and murder of a student nurse in the State hospital where he was confined and subsequently detained as a criminal sexual psychopath. Although John Doe initially provided his consent, the whole process was challenged by a local lawyer, Gabe Kaimowitz,[156] who had heard about the plans to operate on detained patients. Kaimowitz took the Department of Mental Health of the State of Michigan, which would have funded the project, to Court arguing that the operation would violate John Doe's human rights. Upon this intervention, the State withdrew the funding and Drs Rodin and Gottlieb stopped the project. However, the case still went to court, and the court found that "involuntarily detained mental patients cannot give informed and adequate consent to experimental psychosurgical procedures on the brain".[163] This decision by the Michigan Circuit Court goes further than the later recommendations of the National Commission, which did not want to completely exclude detained patients and prisoners from the potential benefits of psychiatric surgery, provided that freedom of consent and the risk/benefit ratio had been independently assessed. However, the Court did allow for the possibility that: "When the state of medical knowledge develops to the extent that the type of psychosurgical intervention proposed here becomes an accepted neurosurgical procedure and is no longer experimental, it is possible, with appropriate review mechanisms, that involuntarily detained mental patients could consent to such an operation."[164]

The Michigan court made another point with potentially far-reaching implications.[163] It referred to the First Amendment to the American Constitution, which protects the freedom of speech: "Congress shall make no law respecting an establishment of religion, or prohibiting the free exercise thereof; or abridging the freedom of speech, or of the press; or the right of the people peaceably to assemble, and to petition the government for a redress of grievances." The court was concerned that psychiatric surgery, by "blunting of emotions" and "deadening of memories" might curb a person's creativity and ability to generate ideas, which were also protected by the First Amendment. The Court explained its reasoning as follows:

> Freedom of speech and expression, and the right of all men to disseminate ideas, popular or unpopular, are fundamental to ordered liberty. Government has no power or right to control man's minds, thoughts, and expressions. This is the command of the First Amendment. And we adhere to it in holding an involuntarily detained mental patient may not consent to experimental psychosurgery. For, if the First Amendment protects the freedom to express ideas, it necessarily follows that it must protect the freedom to generate ideas. Without the latter protection, the former is meaningless.[164]

This argument has implications beyond the application of psychiatric surgery in detained patients or prisoners. Even if a person's ability to consent was not in doubt, one could argue that one cannot ever meaningfully consent (a matter of choice) to a procedure that irreversibly restricted one's own ability to generate ideas (and thus to make choices). In this respect, psychiatric surgery is different from any other type of surgery. However, a libertarian argument can also be made in favour of psychiatric surgery. Valenstein[156] reproduced an editorial in the British broadsheet *The Times* from 2 October 1973 on "Therapy for Criminals".

Regarding brain surgery for uncontrollable sexual impulses, the paper acknowledges the difficulty of obtaining valid consent in prison, especially if the operation is a condition for early release. However, it goes on to argue that "men who ask for treatment to modify their behaviour are not necessarily convicted offenders; and even the critics of such treatments might acknowledge the liberty of an individual to choose it for himself in the absence of any specific pressures from society".

The Michigan court was specifically concerned with amygdalotomy and quoted with some concern the label "sedative neurosurgery" that had been applied by the proponents of this procedure themselves. The court's concern about potentially personality-changing operations, however, would apply more widely. Freeman and Watts had described a clear loss of creative expression in their lobotomised patients:

> they are slow to strive for excellence, are unwilling to drive themselves to better performance, and undertake new forms of artistic expression with great reluctance. The spark may flare up for a brief period after lobotomy, but it is soon extinguished. Patients are apparently not interested in the impractical, the subjective, the impressionistic, the spiritual side of creative art. They have lost the power of imagination...They are simple, direct and uninspired.[82]

Furthermore, the classic leucotomy and lobotomy procedures of the 1940s and 1950s did bring out character features in many patients that they had not exhibited before. Although Sargant and Slater opined that "intelligence is not significantly altered, and alteration in the personality is not likely to take a serious form", in most patients with extensive portions of the frontal lobes destroyed they described the following personality changes:

> After full operations the patient may become demanding in his desires and imperative in their expression. There is a tendency to increased extraversion, which has as its reverse side a lessened capacity for sympathy to others. The patient worries less about the future, and lives much more for the present. He thinks less for himself, becomes more orthodox and matter-of-fact in his view-point. He may become free and easy in his manner, lacking in self-criticism, but willing enough to give opinions on his environment, sometimes so tactlessly as to give offence.[155]

Not unexpectedly, these changes, either towards placidity or towards impulsivity, accompanied by diminished insight and sometimes reduced empathy, are similar to those observed in patients with frontal lobe damage after traumatic brain injury, stroke or tumour. Modern diagnostic classification systems use the term Organic Personality Disorder for such behavioural sequels of brain injury. In a considerable group of patients, thus, psychiatric surgery seems to have replaced one disorder of the mind with another.

4.3   Mind control and society

In the 1970s there was a heated, and by now almost forgotten, debate around the potential role of psychosurgery in the management of violent behaviour. Citing the stunning effects of Delgado's remote brain stimulations on animal behaviour, some proponents of this approach were optimistic that a deeper understanding of the neural roots of violence could open up potential pathways to a treatment that would rid society from a problem that, for many Americans, was the major social issue of their time. In the opposing camp were those who had ideological reservations about research into the brain basis of violence, because it would detract from the more pertinent social and biographical factors; they harboured even more reservations about brain-based intervention because it would open up a path to widespread mind control operations. One extreme expression of the latter camp's views was the 1978 book *The Mind Stealers: Psychosurgery and Mind Control* by the investigative journalist Samuel Chavkin.[163] In its blurb it said, "All over the nation neurosurgeons are now at work modifying or 'curing' drug addicts, alcoholics, homosexuals, neurotics and other 'deviants.'" The actual book then was in large part concerned with surveillance by the state and suspected brainwashing programmes, which were connected with psychiatric surgery only by a hypothetical outlook on how Delgado's stimoceiver devices could potentially be used in this respect, a dystopia which had already featured in Michael Crichton's bestselling novel *Terminal Man* several years earlier, and later in the film remake of *The Manchurian Candidate* with Denzel Washington. Chavkin was particularly critical of the Law Enforcement Assistance Administration, a federal agency that existed from 1968 until 1982, for providing funding for behavioural modification research and suggested that the US prison system was implementing psychiatric surgery particularly to silence politically active prisoners. However, a report in 1974 by the Hastings Center, an independent bioethics centre in the USA, found no evidence of current use of surgical interventions for behaviour control. Admittedly the Hastings Center report was based on the official responses to a survey, and there was still a suspicion in the USA that some states were using surgery for behaviour control in prisons. The report concluded that the Commissioners for Corrections of the US states were instead more interested in expanding a psychotherapeutic approach and behaviour techniques based on a token economy.[165]

At the other extreme to Chavkin's *Mind Stealers* was the highly controversial book *Violence and the Brain* by neurosurgeon Vernon Mark and psychiatrist Frank Ervin. The idea that criminals could be identified by biological features, such as the shape of their face and skull, or indeed certain macroscopic or microscopic changes in their brain, originated in the work of the 19th century Italian psychiatrist and anthropologist Cesare Lombroso. Mark and Ervin wanted to resuscitate Lombroso's basic idea but fill it with substance from their own stimulation studies of the limbic system. Yet, the actual evidence provided in the book for links between specific brain abnormalities and violent behaviour was tenuous and largely based on patients with patent neurological diseases, such as brain tumours or temporal lobe epilepsy, which can occasionally lead to aggressive and violent tendencies in otherwise peaceful individuals. Although these authors are commonly quoted for their suggestion that violence could not only be detected from brain abnormalities but could also be treated by removing these abnormal structures, they were far more circumspect in their actual statements (and largely in their practice as well). Most of the surgery they performed, which normally consisted in the removal of medial parts of the temporal lobes, was actually done on patients with otherwise untreatable temporal lobe epilepsy, where this is an accepted procedure. The main difference from mainstream epilepsy surgery was that they also considered this approach in patients where the main problem was not the clinical severity of the seizures, but its presumed effect on aggressive and violent behaviour. They suggested that electrophysiological abnormalities, especially in the limbic system, might also be detected in some violent individuals without a clinical history of epilepsy and provided some evidence from scalp EEG and depth recordings.[166] However, the specificity of scalp EEG is rather low and the fact that potentials that are also observed during epileptic seizures are seen in the hippocampus during aggressive states, as documented in one of their cases, does not prove that these electrophysiological changes caused the violent behaviour. Although Ervin and Mark implied that surgery might be beneficial against violent tendencies in such individuals, they did not actually put such a programme into practice and their recommendations in *Violence and the Brain* were more about a comprehensive research programme into causes of violent behaviour, incorporating biological and medical assessments, rather than a programme of social engineering. That *Violence and the Brain* could still cause so much controversy at the time shows how shocking the suggestion of a heritable and biologically determined component of violent behaviour was to the proponents of social and environmental causative models almost a hundred years after Cesare Lombroso had first made this suggestion in his book *L'uomo delinquente.*

The immediate clinical application of Ervin and Mark's proposals was stopped when Kaimowitz intervened on behalf of John Doe in the Michigan case discussed above. Rodin and Gottlieb had based the choice of the amygdala as target region for their proposed trial of surgery for sexual aggression on Ervin and Mark's work, largely based on non-sexual aggressive acts in patients with temporal lobe epilepsy (TLE). In fact, if they had proceeded, it is conceivable that they would have produced Klüver-Bucy-type symptoms and thus aggravated rather than alleviated the patient's sexual aggression. However, Mark informed Rodin during the discussions around the John Doe case that, in his view, amygdalotomy for aggressive behaviour was not justified in the absence of evidence of TLE. Rodin, with some justification, thought that Mark had misled the psychiatric community by expressing the view, in *Violence and the Brain,* that abnormal activity in the amygdala could be identified, even in aggressive individuals, without an epilepsy diagnosis.[164] After Mark himself had backtracked on the issue of amygdalotomy for non-epileptic violent offenders the controversy around the surgical route to a "Psychocivilized Society" (Delgado's term) died down. This debate from the 1970s illustrates the dangers of mixing medical, biological and social issues in the absence of sufficient empirical and experimental evidence to link them.

4.4 Illness and conformity

One of the main concerns of the critics of behaviour control programmes was the spectre of Soviet era psychiatry, when diagnoses of mental illness and subsequent detentions in psychiatric hospitals were used to silence dissidents,[85] although this concern did not specifically apply to psychiatric surgery, which had fallen out of favour in the Soviet Union in the 1950s.[167] In their 1982 monograph, O'Callaghan and Carroll also identified a unexpected potential new motivation for control of social deviance by medical means. They argued that the scope of medicine can be defined narrowly as dealing with identifiable diseases, or more broadly as preserving health, which has been defined in the Constitution of the World Health Organisation, drawn up in 1946, as, "a state of complete physical, mental and social well-being and not merely the absence of disease or infirmity."

O'Callaghan & Carroll make the interesting point that by broadening the scope of healthcare in this well-intentioned way one opens up any departure from normality, not just the more narrowly defined diseases, to medical intervention: "While the 'disease' model restricts psychiatric intervention to those fairly circumscribed aspects of human behaviour that can be usefully subsumed by a disease theory, the illness model offers psychiatry unlimited licence".[85] Within this definition, tendencies and behaviours that interfere with a person's social well-being, such as aggression or sexual deviance, could again become targets for surgical intervention, even if they cannot be subsumed under an existing disease model. The opposing view would restrict any medical, and certainly any surgical, intervention to well-defined diseases that have an accepted validity. However, it has to be remembered that psychiatric disease concepts are fluid and rarely supported by "hard", or objective, biological criteria. In the absence of such criteria psychiatry has found it relatively easy to expand its scope by creating new disease categories. The transformation of shyness into a disease, social anxiety, in the course of revising the Diagnostic and Statistical Manual (DSM) of the American Psychiatric Association, is an instructive example of this process.[168] It is much easier to create new diagnostic categories than to remove old ones, because even the less valid diagnoses capture some aspect of patient experience and patients and their clinicians find them helpful as working hypotheses to guide the therapeutic process. The number of diagnoses and the number of people diagnosed with a mental disorder will therefore continue to go up, and the recent, fifth revision of the DSM (DSM5) confirms this trend. Thus, whether we adhere to the WHO's definition of health or to the narrower but ever broadening illness models, the role of psychiatry in modern society will continue to increase.

The scope of medical intervention becomes even broader when it leaves the confines of abnormal or dysfunctional behaviours or traits and is applied to the enhancement of normal behaviour and functions. The most widely cited example of such neuroenhancement is the use of methylphenidate (brand name Ritalin) and other stimulants that activate the dopamine system. Although they are only licensed for properly diagnosed cases of ADHD, the rapid increase in prescriptions over the last 20 years – about 10% of American high school children are now prescribed stimulants – suggests that they are used for behavioural problems in school more generally with the intention of improving academic performance. Increasing use of non-prescribed stimulants for cognitive enhancement by up to 20% of college and university students in the USA has also raised concerns because of the unknown long-term effects of their use and their addictive properties. The potential use of drugs and other interventions originally developed for medical use for such enhancement purposes poses particular problems for medical ethics and legal regulation. For example, risk/benefit ratios are normally evaluated for clinical outcome measures. The same level of scrutiny does not apply to their non-medical use, and thus no formal evidence (from randomised controlled trials) is available to support claims that stimulants actually do enhance academic performance in healthy individuals.

The neurofeedback studies with music students or budding surgeons described in Section 3.2 likewise served the purpose of enhancement rather than the treatment of any disorder. Because they did not involve the use of controlled drugs, and neurofeedback has only minimal side effects, such neuro-enhanced training procedures are probably not contentious. Conversely, invasive procedures for pure enhancement purposes would be far more problematic. The closest comparison in current medical practice might be to injections of botulinum toxin into the skin to treat wrinkles. Botulinum toxin (Botox) is a very potent poison that blocks communication between nerve cells and thus aids muscle relaxation. By analogy, someone who is unhappy not with their looks but with their intelligence could ask a surgeon to insert a DBS electrode to improve their intellectual power. At present the risk of side effects may be considered too high but present-day cosmetic surgery is not without risks either. If cosmetic surgery of the skin and subcutaneous tissues is ethically acceptable, the same principles should apply to enhancement procedures if they are performed on the brain. Those who are bothered by the prospect of such cosmetic neurosurgery do not need to worry too much, though, because it is unlikely that such procedures will become available any time soon. So far, DBS has not produced expert musicians or surgeons and none of the many procedures of psychiatric surgery has provided any evidence to suggest that it may be suitable for cognitive enhancement. Thus, like the speculations about widespread use of psychiatric surgery to control violence in the 1970s, today's debate about brain stimulators for enhancement may remain within the realm of science fiction.

4.5   Social myopia: exclusive focus on organic causes?

Very few people would doubt that mental illness has both biological and social roots, but individual psychiatrists (and patients) differ in the amount of weight they put on one or the other. The general tendencies within psychiatry have also oscillated between the two poles of biological and social determinism since the beginnings of scientific psychiatry in the mid-19th century. The second half of the 19th century was characterised by a belief in the ability of biological techniques, such as the microscopic examination of brain tissue after a patient's death, to reveal the causes of mental illness. This brain-based model paved the way for early experiments in psychiatric surgery by Burckhardt and Puusepp, and for its continuation in the lobotomy programmes of the mid-20th century. For a certain time, this biological model coexisted with the psychoanalytical model introduced by Sigmund Freud, which emphasised the importance of early childhood experience for the development of depression, anxiety and compulsive symptoms, collectively labelled as neuroses. Although the causal models of psychoanalysis had little empirical foundation this movement created sensitivity to the role of biographical factors and family life in the development of mental illness. However, the psychoanalytical theorists were shockingly myopic when it came to the real-life traumatic experiences of their (female) patients. It took several decades to recognise the important role of actual sexual trauma as a risk factor for later mental health problems.[169] By the middle of the 20th century most American outpatient psychiatry, dealing with neuroses and other less severe cases, was dominated by psychoanalysis, whereas the biological model survived in the asylums and facilitated the rapid uptake of lobotomy. The second wave of biological psychiatry, which was triggered by the discovery of effective antipsychotic and antidepressant drugs in the 1950s, soon swept lobotomy away but it also massively curtailed the influence of psychoanalysis.[170] Any psychiatric surgery is founded on the assumption that neural processes are pivotal for mental illness and thus predicated on a biological model. After the success of pharmacological therapies in the 1960s the next main boost for the new biological psychiatry came in the 2000s with the discovery of the first genetic variants that are associated with common mental disorders. This revived belief in biological causation in psychiatry may have contributed to the renewed interest in neuromodulation, although biological psychiatry has, so far, not contributed any biomarkers that could serve as targets for intervention. Such a focus on organic remedies is not necessarily wrong, provided it can be shown that they work. After all, the situation is essentially the same for neuromodulation as for the widely prescribed psychiatric drugs. They may be very effective but they cannot be regarded as causal treatments in the strict sense. This entails a risk, particularly for the irreversible treatments. If, at a later stage, the true cause of a mental illness is discovered it may be too late to attack it because the surgery has irreversibly damaged some other functions. Even worse, surgery (and drug therapy entails the same risk) could become an alternative to a remediation of the patient's personal circumstances and thus serve to prolong oppressive social relations. Psychosurgeons in previous generations were rather matter-of-fact about such scenarios. A case report by the British surgeon Geoffrey Knight, who invented stereotactic subcaudate tractotomy in 1961, exemplifies this myopia for social circumstances:

> a woman of 38 had suffered from tension and anxiety since childhood; at 19 following marriage to a sadist she developed multiple jerks and sweating so severe that she had to change her clothes several times a day and obsessional tidiness and depression also developed. Following operation 10 years ago she was immediately dramatically improved; within 2 months the jerking, sweating and suicidal impulses were gone, she was able to put things away in the wardrobe and forget all about abnormal tidiness.... She has maintained this complete improvement.[171]

The psychiatrists Sargant and Slater were even more upfront about the anti-progressive elements in psychosurgery[155] when they singled out "the reactive depression in which environmental factors of an irremediable kind are involved" as potentially responsive to leucotomy:

> A depressed woman, for instance, may owe her illness to a psychopathic husband who cannot change and will not accept treatment. Separation might be the answer, but is ruled out by other ties such as children, by the patient's financial or emotional dependence, or by her religious views. In such cases, which may be very intractable, we have seen patients enabled to return to the difficult environment and cope with it in a way which had hitherto been impossible.

Of course, the widespread practice of prescribing benzodiazepines or other tranquillisers in such cases is equally anti-progressive and almost as difficult to reverse (because of the addictive potential of these drugs), but surgery to make a woman compliant with an abusive husband comes dangerously close to social control.

The Australian moral philosopher John Kleinig, who had a generally favourable attitude to psychiatric surgery, acknowledged that critics of this field feared a:

> dehumanisation of social life...Psychosurgery is seen as just one more step in the direction of "Brave New World", in which genuinely human agonies and frustrations are blotted out by "soma", and replaced by something which is comfortable but not a genuinely human happiness and satisfaction. The problems remain but they no longer trouble.[172]

The cases of the unfortunate women cited above show that this fear was not entirely unfounded.

4.6 Preventive surgery?

Sexual offenders pose a considerable risk of reoffending. Most estimates for the long-term risk of committing another sexual offence range between 10% and 20%, and risk predictions in individual cases have a large margin of error. Psychological interventions do not seem to reduce this risk appreciably,[173] and the effects of anti-androgen treatments are difficult to assess.[174] Even surgical castration, which is arguably the most radical treatment available and whose application in detained individuals has been criticised on human rights grounds, provides no absolute protection against reoffending because the sexual interest can be reinstated with testosterone replacement. The dearth of valid prediction tools and effective treatment options has created a major conundrum for legislators. Should sexual offenders be released from prison when they have served their term and be a risk to the community? Or should they be detained as long as they pose a risk – and thus potentially indefinitely – which would result in a detention term disproportionate to the original offence? Over the last 25 years legislatures and courts, for example in 20 states of the USA, several Australian provinces, Germany, Scotland and England have increasingly favoured the second option.[175, 176] Although legal principles forbid disproportionate punishment and multiple convictions for the same crime (under the principle of double jeopardy), such confinement has been justified on the grounds of its preventive and rehabilitative function. In the USA, all state laws providing for confinement of sexually violent predators (SVP) follow the criteria set out by the Supreme Court in the case of Kansas v. Hendricks (1997). In order to be legally detained in a special facility beyond the term of the original conviction the offender needs to have:

(1) a history of sexually harmful behavior; (2) a mental abnormality that produces an impairment of control over sexually harmful behavior; (3) a prediction of future sexually dangerous behavior.[175]

For example, the Community Protection Act of the State of Washington defines a sexually violent predator as "any person who has been convicted of or charged with a crime of sexual violence and who suffers from a mental abnormality or personality disorder which makes the person likely to engage in predatory acts of sexual violence if not confined in a secure facility" (www.doc.wa.gov/community/sex offenders/civilcommitment.asp; accessed on 4 August 2013). This confinement, which has to be ordered by a court and is subject to annual review, serves the purposes of "control, care, and treatment". Because of the low effectiveness of existing treatments and the high margin of error of risk prediction (with experts preferring to err on the side of caution), these provisions have resulted in thousands of detentions, without much prospect of release.[175]

How would someone who is confined under such an SVP law in the USA or elsewhere look at the option of psychiatric surgery? What if they read some of the positive case reports from the 1960s and 1970s and found the prospect of a hypothalamotomy, which might reduce their sex drive, attractive even if only as a means of moving into the lower-risk category that would be eligible for supervision in a less restrictive setting. A court following the principles of the Michigan court that adjudicated the John Doe case might tell him that he cannot provide truly free consent to such a procedure because of the coercion implied in his confinement. However, he might disagree and argue that it is very reasonable for him to opt for an operation with relatively low medical risk that would increase his chance of release over the almost certain prospect of lifelong confinement. This legal challenge has not been made yet, partly because this type of operation is currently not offered by neurosurgeons, but it would be interesting to see how a present-day court would respond to this moral and legal challenge.

Another reason why this scenario is currently hypothetical is that we lack formal evidence about the effectiveness of hypothalamotomy in relapse prevention and that it would be very difficult to obtain such evidence in SVP. It is almost a Catch-22 problem; the effectiveness of the procedure can only be tested if perpetrators are released into the community, but courts would only order a release into the community if the operation is proven to be effective. However, if there was a general agreement amongst surgeons, specialists in sexual disorders and the legal profession that neurosurgery should be offered for patients with paraphilias that predispose to sexual offending, for example paedophilia, its effectiveness could be tested in patients before they actually offend. Because the expectations for psychosocial interventions to reduce sexual offending have not been fulfilled so far it might now be time to leave behind the ideological battlegrounds of the 1970s and engage in a new debate on the role of psychiatric surgery in the treatment and prevention of sexual aggression.

In recent years the ethical debate seems to have shifted towards a more pragmatic approach that is not exclusively concerned with the protection from real or perceived coercion but also recognises the human right to have access to treatments that can potentially alleviate suffering or improve rehabilitative prospects. A group of European ethicists, neurosurgeons and psychiatrists who investigated current issues in brain stimulation and related procedures in relation to another mental illness whose sufferers often come into conflict with the law, concluded:

> Should a brain-invasive treatment for severe psychopathy ever become available, subject to common criteria for weighing the potential risks against the potential benefits of this procedure, then nothing stands in the way of offering such a treatment to people in preventive detention if that is the only alternative to their being kept in custody indefinitely.... We hold that, in such a situation, the state would be not only entitled but even obliged to make the respective offer for the following reasons. Having a brain-invasive treatment for psycho-/sociopathy in order to regain one's status as a free person might be less burdensome to that person than an indefinite detention.[177]

4.7   Ethics of DBS

Early human brain stimulation experiments shared the widespread public condemnation of lobotomy. Heath described intense negative reactions from the scientific community and accusations of mind control and manipulation. He retorted that:

> In sharp contrast to the "mind control" that can result from interpersonal therapy, use of addictive drugs, and membership in certain

cults, it was never possible to control the mind with our techniques, nor was that our intent.[47]

Although Heath was doubtless right about the mind control that can be exerted by cults, drugs and even psychotherapists who deviate from professional standards, his critics may also have had a point. With some of his behaviour-changing interventions, notably the induction of rage, it is difficult to see what the intended long-term therapeutic effect may have been. Moreover, the ability to stimulate a specific brain site and thus evoke a specific memory and an immediate associated emotional state may still be more powerful than what can be achieved with purely psychological techniques. Some of his protocols were clearly ethically problematic, notably the attempt to recondition a 24-year old homosexual man by pairing septal stimulation with movie scenes showing heterosexual intercourse, as recounted by Valenstein.[44] However, when it comes to fundamentally altering someone's character and moral fabric, history knows of ways and means that are more effective than anything that has so far been achieved through brain stimulation.

Compared to the brain stimulation experiments of the middle of the 20th century, the new wave of psychiatric DBS with chronically implanted electrodes has had a much more positive reception. It has not encountered the critique levelled against destructive surgery and has largely been accepted as a potentially useful treatment of last resort for depression and OCD, although it rests on a smaller evidence base than stereotactic lesion techniques. For example, a recent survey of press coverage of new neurostimulation techniques for neurological and psychiatric disorders in the USA and the UK found an overwhelmingly positive attitude. Only 4% of articles had a critical tone, and ethical issues such as resource allocation and patient autonomy did not feature prominently.[178] This is in striking contrast not only to the coverage of psychiatric surgery but also to that of the most established psychiatric neurostimulation technique, ECT, which has polarised opinion almost as much as lobotomy.

We can only speculate about the reasons for the positive response to DBS. To some extent, psychiatric DBS might have ridden the wave of neurological DBS, where there is little dispute about its usefulness in Parkinson's disease and other movement disorders. Although DBS studies have targeted the same pathways as older lesion techniques they have adduced modern neuroimaging to identify putative pathological nodes and thus to provide the underlying biological model with the scientific credibility many of the older surgical approaches had been lacking. In principle, DBS also offers the option of closed loop systems, where the stimulation is adjusted to fluctuations in pathological neural activity. It could also potentially be adjusted by the patients themselves, although this might bring therapeutic DBS dangerously close to self-stimulation experiments. Adjustment of stimulation strength or frequency on the basis of clinical effects is more realistic for some neurological conditions than for current psychiatric applications, where clinical effects take weeks to arise. Finally, DBS is, in principle, reversible and thus does not come with the burden of irreversible destruction of healthy tissue. Unlike destructive surgery, which is always likely to be a treatment of last resort, DBS might thus at some point be considered at even earlier stages of the disease process (drawing on recent experience with PD), although this would probably require a better understanding of the biological processes leading to the psychiatric disorder in question.

However, psychiatric DBS as currently practised does share several features with stereotactic destructive surgery. It uses preset stimulation parameters that are supposed to inhibit the same pathways that are lesioned in cingulotomy or capsulotomy procedures. Because stimulation is normally continued over years, it probably introduces lasting changes in the affected neural pathways. Whether these are negative or positive for brain function is essentially unknown.[159] Sudden deterioration of the patient's mental state has been reported in cases of stimulator malfunction or in cases in which stimulation was discontinued as part of the clinical trial protocol. It is thus unknown whether psychiatric DBS is truly reversible.

Unless DBS turns out to be more effective than stereotactic lesions there may be arguments favouring the latter from both a medical and an ethical point of view. Even if surgical complication rates are roughly similar, lesion surgery is likely to have fewer long-term side effects because it does not involve long-term implantation of foreign material. Furthermore, DBS entails a commitment by the medical team to long-term surgical and psychiatric aftercare. This is a major task to take on and has so far only been achieved in well-resourced academic centres in the context of clinical trials. Any team undertaking DBS needs to address the issue of aftercare beyond the duration of the trial. Along similar lines and all else being equal, lesion surgery has lower long-term costs and thus would make fewer demands on already stretched healthcare budgets and be more realistic to roll out in low-income countries. Considerations of resource allocation thus come down in favour of cingulotomy or capsulotomy over DBS. At the same time, relief of depression or OCD through destructive surgery may come at the cost of memory problems, personality changes and an increasing apathy and fatigue. The chapter on the ethics of psychiatric surgery in a recent standard textbook on stereotactic neurosurgery very reasonably called for head-to-head comparisons of DBS against established lesion procedures in order to allow for a formal appreciation of the risk/ benefit ratios and costs of the different procedures.[179] Yet the current trend, at least in Europe and the USA, favours replacing lesion surgery with DBS without conducting formal comparisons beforehand, and extending the indication of DBS to all disorders that had historically been in the purview of psychosurgery, with the notable exception of sexual disorders.

Some of the psychiatric applications of DBS may even bypass the need for rigorous clinical trials. In 2009, the Food and Drug Administration (FDA) of the USA granted Medtronic, one of the main manufacturers of electrodes for DBS, a humanitarian device exemption for the use of one of its devices for treatment-refractory OCD. A humanitarian device exemption (HDE) is intended to allow patients with uncommon conditions access to new treatments that may be difficult to test in formal trials. Normally, such devices or other treatments whose effectiveness has not been proven can only be used in the context of clinical trials (in this case, a new medical device requires an investigational device exemption). Under a HDE, however, a medical device can be used in clinical practice without prior demonstration of its effectiveness. Although this process may speed up the dissemination of promising treatments to patients with rare and desperate conditions, it has rightly been questioned whether it was justified in the case of OCD which, after all, is a condition affecting several million Americans, several hundred thousands of whom do not respond to currently available treatments.[180] Such a HDE may be attractive to manufacturers in the short-term because it gives them access to new patient groups, but stifles research into the clinical effects and mechanisms of the intervention (and may ultimately even reduce its uptake in clinical practice). Because in its current state of development psychiatric DBS should be confined to appropriately equipped and specialised academic centres anyway, it would make perfect sense to restrict its use to formal clinical trials until better evidence about its effects and side effects has been accumulated.

DBS for movement disorders also brings up ethical issues, in addition to general considerations of consent and patient safety. Reports of suicides by PD patients on DBS, even after favourable neurological outcomes, have caused concerns. It is still not entirely clear whether suicide rates on DBS are higher than those in the general PD patient population and if so, how this might be explained. In addition to direct effects of DBS on limbic pathways psychosocial factors may also need to be considered:

> DBS has revolutionized the management of PD and it often has a profound effect on individuals and their families. Often having to rely on others for basic needs, many patients regain much of their independence following DBS surgery, which may require significant psychosocial adjustment. Many patients find it difficult to view themselves outside of the sick role as many aspects of their life had been devoted to coping with their disease.[181]

Such considerations reinforce the need for long-term monitoring of DBS patients, whatever their diagnosis, not just for the correct functioning of the electronics but also for any impact of the procedure on their mental health and general well-being.

4.8   DBS in patients who are unable to provide consent

Even patients with normal cognitive functions may be restricted in their capacity to provide free consent to DBS and other psychiatric surgery procedures, for example because they are suffering from a desperate illness and have unrealistic hopes (in which case careful explanations of the risks and expected benefits are needed) or because they are in the criminal justice system and may associate consent to the procedure with the hope of early release. Yet DBS might also be considered for patients who, by the very nature of their disorder, do not have the cognitive capacity to provide consent. The relevant patient groups here are those with severe intellectual impairment and aggressive behaviour and patients in vegetative or minimally conscious states. As discussed in Chapter 1, after the patient has spent a certain time in VS or MCS, recovery becomes extremely unlikely. DBS has therefore been tried to increase wakefulness and communication in these patients. Medtronic even sponsored a large trial with about 50 patients in VS who received electrical stimulation of thalamic nuclei or the cervical spinal cord. The results of this trial, which included Terri (Theresa) Schiavo, the VS patient who later became famous worldwide because of the legal battle around her right to die, were disappointing. However, some investigators promote the potential use of thalamic DBS for MCS, where brain damage may not be as widespread as in VS and the chance of benefiting from the stimulation of thalamo-cortical circuits may be higher.

The basis for this suggestion is from a case study of a patient in MCS who received bilateral stimulation to the central thalamus. This patient was still totally dependent on 24-hour care but improved in his ability to utter words and eat during periods of stimulation.[182] Although this may seem a small benefit for an invasive procedure we do not know what effect this very limited gain of function may have had on patient's quality of life.

The medical ethicist Joseph Fins has suggested specific safeguarding procedures for DBS in such patients with "decisional incapacity".[183] It is well-established ethical and legal practice to obtain surrogate consent for medical procedures for patients who cannot make such decisions for themselves. Persons making these decisions for the patient, for example close relatives or other legal representatives, are expected to act in the patient's best interest and to take his or her presumed will into account as much as possible. Even decisions about established medical procedures that entail a certain risk or discomfort may not be easy under these circumstances, but what about consent to enter a clinical trial for a risky procedure with uncertain benefits, such as DBS? Fins suggested that inclusion in such trials should require the consensus of the patient's legal representative, the patient's clinician, the investigator leading the trial and an independent patient advocate. He considered the alternative of completely excluding patients without decisional capacity from trials of new, risky but potentially beneficial procedures to be unethical because patients not only had a right to be protected from harm but also to have access to new treatments:

> Although all involved in research have the duty to protect the incapacitated subject from harm, the principles of respect for persons, beneficence and justice can also be invoked to assert a fiduciary obligation to design and execute well-considered and scientifically sound clinical trials for this historically marginalized population.[120]

4.9 Ethics of BCIs

The need to raise realistic expectations is also important for decisions on implantation of electrode grids for BCIs. Although patients with high spinal injuries or brainstem lesions, for whom this procedure might be considered, generally have preserved cognitive function, their capacity for realistic assessment of the risks and benefits of such an invasive procedure may be skewed by the desperate nature of their illness and their high level of disability. At the same time, this means that, after careful consideration, they may be willing to take on the risks of neuro-surgery, even for benefits that may seem relatively small to observers, for example being able to point at objects or pick letters from a computer screen, because that would make a major difference to their interaction with the outside world and thus their quality of life. However, one would need to assess carefully in each individual case whether their other preserved output modalities (such as verbalisations, facial movements) could be used to train signal detection algorithms to obtain similar levels of prosthesis control without the need for surgical implantation of sensors. Conversely, it is unlikely that non-invasive EEG will take over this function in the near future because at present EEG-based BCIs are largely confined to binary communication, similar to Jean-Dominique Bauby's blink responses.

Even such relatively simple communication devices could be crucial in allowing patients to communicate and express their views, including those on future medical intervention. Although neurofeedback training for BCI control can be stressful to the patient it is reasonable to assume a general interest on the part of the patient to learn a strategy that enables them to express their thoughts and wishes. Furthermore, if the fMRI decoding techniques described in Section 1.6 can be developed into a communication device for locked-in patients that does not require lengthy training, it can be used to ask patients for their consent to engage with any brain reading procedure. It would be preferable if patients were in a position to express consent in some way before the scanning process is started, but this is obviously not possible in some locked-in patients and in all patients with VS or MCS. Privacy issues are also important. After all, the scans may not only reveal whether a patient experiences pain or not (although the technology is not yet mature enough to make such inferences) or whether they can imagine moving their left or right arms but they may also allow investigators to decode the patient's thoughts unbeknownst to the patients themselves. Although this is presently only a theoretical possibility, the potential of brain imaging to read patient's minds needs to be taken into account when making decisions about diagnostic brain reading in unresponsive or uncommunicative patients.[29]

Recent high profile cases in the UK, for example that of Tony Nicklinson, who unsuccessfully campaigned for his right to die after a stroke left him in an incomplete locked-in state, have flagged up the conflict between the wishes of some paralysed patients to be helped to die (with considerable public support), and the legal position that gener-ally forbids this. What is unknown at present is whether, once severely disabled, completely locked-in patients have access to BCI communication devices, there will be increasing numbers of patients expressing a wish for assisted dying. Tony Nicklinson died on 22 August 2012, shortly after he had lost his High Court case to allow doctors to help him end his life. According to a statement from the family, he refused to take any food after he lost his legal battle.

4.10 Ethics of neurofeedback

Neurofeedback poses far fewer safety concerns than surgical intervention. Experiences from over one hundred participants so far has indicated that fMRI-NF is well tolerated,[142] and the experience of thousands of patients who underwent EEG-NF did not bring up concerns about major side effects either. The risk profile is rather similar to that of psychotherapy. Patients may find the training procedure stressful or be frustrated by their inability to gain control over their brain activation. This problem can be addressed to some extent by gradual learning or shaping procedures, whereby the difficulty of the task is progressively adjusted to the patient's performance to ensure consistent levels of positive feedback. In cases where the training is successful and the mental states induced are experienced as particularly pleasant and rewarding, patients may become accustomed to the boost from their regular neurofeedback sessions and may even become psychologically dependent. This risk can be addressed by structured homework exercises that allow patients to practice self-regulation and associated mental strategies at home, without the need for regular MRI scans.

Nevertheless, fMRI-NF similar to other high-tech procedures introduced in this book (DBS, stereotactic surgery, BCIs) requires access to expensive equipment, which puts a strain on the resources of publicly funded healthcare systems (or on the funds of the patients if they have to pay privately). As with any expensive medical treatment there are always ways of spending the funds on lower cost interventions that benefit a wider group of people, for example vaccinations or public health programmes. However, such resource comparisons are generally theoretical in nature and high-technology and high-cost interventions for small numbers of otherwise treatment-refractory patients should not be pitched against lower cost preventive medicine. It is necessary to allocate resources to both types of medicine. Furthermore, high-cost interventions may ultimately decrease in price, especially if take-up increases or lower cost transfer technologies are found. One such scenario for neurofeedback would be that only a few initial scanning sessions would be required before the training can be transferred onto ambulatory monitoring devices, such as EEG caps or smartphones. Finally, high-tech interventions that give patients back their quality of life and save healthcare costs elsewhere, for example by reducing the need for inpatient treatment, can be very cost effective. Evaluation of the health economics should accompany studies of neurofeedback and other brain control interventions, but the cost of the procedure and equipment alone should certainly not deter from further developments in this field.

Neurofeedback is an attractive addition to the currently available psychological and behavioural interventions in mental health because it puts the patient in the driving seat: "In a sense, NFB enables a subject to have a greater degree of control of brain activity mediating certain perceptions and behaviors than DBS or BCIs."[184] Although in most cases it will probably be complementary to other, more established interventions, it may also become an alternative for the considerable number of patients who are reluctant to hand over control over their mental processes to a drug or a therapist.

4.11 Outlook

The debates charted in this book are beset with artificial dichotomies: neurology vs. psychiatry; defined pathological targets vs. cutting healthy tissue; reversible brain stimulation vs. irreversible lesions; autonomy vs. surgical mind control; to name but a few. However, the morality of therapeutic brain intervention is rarely as clear cut as these divisions may suggest.

Although neurological diseases are generally well-defined, those without a unitary genetic cause or clear biomarkers can be as difficult to diagnose as psychiatric disorders. Parkinson's disease is one example and although the target areas for DBS, unlike those for depression or OCD, have been determined through animal models, the mechanisms that bring about its clinical effects are as obscure in the neurological as in the psychiatric disorders. Furthermore, in all clinical applications of DBS, whether for chronic pain, movement disorders or mental health, a large part of the evidence for clinical effects is based on subjective measures (e.g. pain ratings, quality of life questionnaires, depression scales) rather than objective physiological parameters.

The reversibility of DBS is often quoted as an advantage over irreversible lesion surgery, but the situation may not be that simple. On the one hand, the long-term changes after surgery, which can be positive or negative, suggest that compensatory circuits can form after focal surgery in white matter. On the other hand, neural circuits adapt to long-term deep brain stimulation, and it is unknown whether an electrode can be simply removed after many years of stimulation without ill effects (the experience from occasional battery failures suggests otherwise) or whether patients may even become addicted to DBS. Finally, although DBS and surgical interventions seem to require the patient to hand over control over their brain to a surgeon, some ethicists have argued that invasive interventions can also enable patients to regain autonomy in cases where their initiative and volition have been severely impaired by their mental disorder.[184]

As a result of these dichotomies the current public debate is marked by a striking dissociation between enthusiastic support for the promising therapeutic potential of DBS, especially for neurological disorders, and the condemnation of lesion surgery, especially if applied to behavioural disorders. Yet the ethical principles governing DBS and lesion surgery are not fundamentally different. Furthermore, on what basis are the more behavioural disorders, such as opiate addiction, less appropriate for invasive interventions than the more classic neurological disorders, such as Parkinson's disease? Both can be chronically disabling and progressive and patients are only considered for surgery if they do not respond sufficiently to multiple standard interventions. Denying patients with behavioural disorders access to invasive therapies (assuming they can be shown to be effective) that are granted as a matter of course to neurological patients, entails the risk of further increasing the stigma associated with psychiatric illness.

It is possible to define certain interventions that are clearly not permissible, for example the leucotomies performed on the women mentioned in Section 4.5 who became depressed because they were suffering under sadistic husbands. No medical intervention can be justified if its primary aim is to make the patient compliant with a social situation that could be changed otherwise. Here the moral imperative is to change the norms and reality of a society rather than the brains of the people who suffer under them. There is another group of interventions that should only be performed under strict legal safeguards and transparent, international medical evaluation. This group includes operations on minors, patients without the capacity to consent and detained patients, as well as invasive interventions for addiction and sexual disorders. One reason for the more restrictive approach to these conditions is that the potential for perceived coercion is higher than in depression or OCD because many patients would have been in conflict with the law at some point. Even if no such link is made officially patients may be under the impression that consent to an operation would have a positive effect on their legal proceedings. Another reason is that the published evidence for the effectiveness of these procedures (e.g. hypothalamotomy to reduce sex drive, destruction of the nucleus accumbens to promote abstinence) comes from individual groups or small numbers of centres and they cannot be regarded as internationally established. Yet, even the more established lesion approaches (capsulotomy and cingulotomy for depression and OCD) and emerging DBS protocols targeting related pathways should only be performed in the context of prospective studies, ideally in a formal trial setting with a control group (for example, comparing one of the lesion approaches with DBS or in waiting list designs). The two main reasons for this requirement are, firstly, that regardless of the relatively high numbers of patients who have received stereotactic lesions over the last six decades the evidence base is still too thin for a proper evaluation of its effectiveness; and, secondly, that the available evidence indicates that a certain proportion of patients respond well to surgery, whereas other patients do not respond at all. It is always useful in clinical medicine to have data from prospective studies that allow the identification of markers for future treatment response. This is particularly true for invasive interventions where, if non-responders can be identified beforehand, the mortality and morbidity (side effects) associated with the operation can be avoided. Because the numbers of psychiatric patients for any individual functional neurosurgery unit are low these studies should occur in multi-centre collaborations. The clinicaltrials. gov database lists several clinical trials of DBS in depression, but most of these have 20 or fewer patients and would clearly benefit from more coordination. The humanitarian device exemption granted for DBS in OCD by the American Food and Drugs Administration was almost certainly premature and it is encouraging to see that the pioneers in this field are not intending to acquiesce to this decision but move the clinical evaluation of DBS effects forward.

Because of the strict criteria for patient selection psychiatric DBS is likely to remain a procedure for small numbers of patients, even if these future clinical trials corroborate the positive clinical effects. Conversely, neurofeedback, which has a much lower threshold for patient inclusion, could become a technique that is rolled out in parallel with other patient training and education programmes on a larger scale, and even started in early stages of the disease process. Such an application of (EEG-)neurofeedback is already established for ADHD in some countries. Because it is still not clear whether its effects are superior to placebo or control interventions, health systems with a relatively strict commissioning policy based on criteria of evidence-based medicine, like the UK's National Health Service, are unlikely to adopt it. However, from an ethical point of view it is probably acceptable to offer an intervention that has no, or minimal, side effects and improves a patient's level of functioning and well-being, even if it mainly (or exclusively) harnesses placebo effects. In relation to neurofeedback with fMRI, the next five years will show whether the considerable international interest within the research and clinical communities can be converted into tangible clinical benefits in studies of depression, Parkinson's disease, addiction, post-traumatic stress disorder and other neurological and psychiatric disorders. Neurofeedback with fMRI is initially much more expensive to run than EEG neurofeedback or simple biofeedback. One way of delivering it in practice may be to set up neurorehabilitation centres that incorporate a scanning unit for both diagnostic and therapeutic purposes and also provide transfer technologies, such as gaming consoles for motor feedback and virtual reality rooms for feedback on visual imagery and social interaction.

Over the centuries people have tried to control the brain through three different avenues: by interaction at the level of mental processes (for example, education and psychotherapy); through modification or modulation of the brain itself (for example, psychiatric surgery and neurofeedback); and through interaction with the body (for example, biofeedback or physical exercise). Clinical experience shows that it is very difficult, if not impossible, to create lasting, positive changes by using just one of these avenues. In order to benefit increasing numbers of people with mental or neurological illnesses modern brain control will therefore need to incorporate psychological and physical training as well. This limitation is also an opportunity because it implies that brain control will not be a completely passive affair but one where the patients themselves get a chance to take control of their own brains, bodies and minds.

Glossary

Amygdala: Group of nuclei (accumulations of neurons) located in front of the hippocampus. Amongst its main functions is the learning of emotional responses.

Amygdalotomy: Removal of the amygdala on one side (unilateral) or both (bilateral).

Amyotrophic lateral sclerosis (ALS): A neurodegenerative disorder that leads to progressive loss of motor neurons in the brain and spinal cord. American baseball legend Lou Gehrig was a prominent sufferer, and ALS is also known as "Lou Gehrig's disease", particularly in the USA.

Angiogram: A way of imaging blood vessels with x-ray by injecting a contrast medium into the blood.

Anorexia nervosa: Eating disorder, characterised by low body mass index, food restriction and/or over-exercising.

Atrial fibrillation: A heart condition with irregular and often abnormally fast heart rate.

Bed nucleus of the stria terminalis (BNST): A part of the extended amygdala region, implicated in fear responses and addiction. Its central division in sexually dimorphic: it is larger in men than women.

Body mass index (BMI): Quotient of weight (in kg) over height (squared, in m^2). Values between 18.5 and 25 are considered to be in the normal range.

Brain computer interface (BCI): A circuit that enables signals from the brain to control an output device, for example a computer cursor or a robot.

Capsulotomy (internal): Lesioning of the anterior limb of the internal capsule, normally by stereotactic means (local application of heat through an electrode). The anterior limb of the internal capsule carries

thalamo-frontal fibres, including the medial forebrain bundle. The
posterior limb carries the cortico-spinal (pyramidal) motor tract, and
thus lesions to it would result in loss of motor function.

Caudate nucleus: Part of the basal ganglia adjacent to the lateral ventricles. Forms their main input station.

Cingulate gyrus: The part of the medial frontal lobe above the corpus
callosum. Liaison station between "higher" cortical areas and the
limbic system.

Cingulotomy: Lesion of the cingulate gyrus/cingulum.

Cingulum: White matter bundle between corpus callosum and cingulate gyrus. Its posterior part connects with the hippocampus.

Computed tomography (CT): An extension of the x-ray technique that
uses computer processing to obtain tomographic images (virtual slices
through the body).

Continuous performance task (CPT): A psychological test that probes
the integrity of attention and response control.

Cortex, cortical: The cerebral cortex is the sheet of gray matter covering
the hemispheres of the brain. It contains most of the neurons of the
hemispheres (the others are in the basal ganglia). In adults it is about
2mm–4mm thick and has three to six layers, characterised by different
cell composition. Most human cortex is neocortex (thus new in evolutionary terms), which has six layers.

Deep Brain Stimulation (DBS): Application of current to an area of the
brain through a (normally stereotactically inserted) electrode. "Deep"
refers to areas that are not on the cortical surface.

Depression: A mood disorder, characterised through (often recurrent)
episodes of abnormal sadness, lack of motivation, inability to experience joy and somatic symptoms, such as sleep disturbance, fatigue,
loss of appetite or loss of libido.

Diencephalon: The part of the brain below the hemispheres, mainly
contains the thalamus and hypothalamus.

Dorsolateral prefrontal cortex (DLPFC): Part of the frontal lobe,
involved in working memory and executive functions.

Electrical stimulation of the brain (ESB): A summary term for DBS and
stimulation of areas at the surface of the brain.

Electroconvulsive therapy (ECT): A treatment for depression that
induces seizures through high-intensity transcranial electrical stimulation. It is also used for rare complications of schizophrenia.

Electroencephalography (EEG): Recording of electrical activity from the brain through the intact skull by means of electrodes. Developed by Hans Berger in the 1920s.

Electronarcosis: A historical treatment of schizophrenia that entailed the induction of coma of several minutes duration through high-intensity transcranial electrical stimulation.

Encephalitis: Inflammation of the brain. It can be caused by infectious agents or by autoimmune processes occurring when the patient's own immune system attacks cells in the brain.

Essential tremor (ET): A common movement disorder characterised by prominent tremor during voluntary movements.

Frontal lobe: Most anterior part of a brain hemisphere. It issupposed to have developed most in evolutionary terms (e.g. it is proportionally much larger in humans compared to the rest of the brain, than even in great apes). Contains areas of motor control, memory, decision making, cognitive control and emotion regulation.

Functional magnetic resonance imaging (fMRI): Technique to record vascular signals from the brain, which allows for drawing inferences on the underlying neural activity.

Functional near infrared spectroscopy (fNIRS): Technique to record changes in blood oxygenation from superficial areas in the brain by shining light of specific wave length through the skull.

Globus pallidus (internal) (GPi): A part of the basal ganglia, involved in motor control, and one of the target areas of DBS for movement disorders.

Grey matter: Accumulation of neurons in sheets (cortex) or lumps (nuclei).

Hamilton Depression Rating Scale (HDRS): The HDRS assesses depressive symptoms with 17 items. Higher scores correspond to more severe depression. A score of seven or less generally denotes remission from depression. The HDRS is often used to assess the effects of treatments for depression.

Hippocampus: Area of evolutionarily old, three-layered cortex in the medial temporal lobe. Crucial for memory encoding and retrieval.

Humanitarian device exemption (HDE): An exemption granted by the U.S. Food and Drug Administration that allows manufacturers to market medical devices for specific rare conditions although its effectiveness has not been demonstrated.

Hypothalamotomy: Lesion of the hypothalamus, most commonly its ventromedial nucleus (in German operations on sexual offenders) or posterior medial part (Sano's operations for aggressive behaviour).

Hypothalamus: Part of the diencephalon. Central control station for the hormone system and bodily homoeostasis (balance of metabolic processes).

Impulse control disorders: A group of behavioural disorders defined by the inability to resist relatively specific and isolated impulses, including kleptomania (impulse to steal), pyromania (impulse to set fire), pathological gambling (impulse to gamble) and trichotillomania (impulse to pull out one's hair).

Insulin coma therapy: A historical treatment for schizophrenia that involved injecting the patient with insulin to induce coma through depriving the brain of glucose, often on several days in succession.

Klüver Bucy syndrome: A symptom complex comprising problems with memory and visual recognition of objects, increased libido, overeating and the compulsory tendency to put things in the mouth ("hyperorality"). It arises after bilateral destructions of the amygdala and was first described by psychologist Heinrich Klüver and neurosurgeon Paul Bucy in monkeys, although it can also occur in humans.

Limbic system: Group of cortical areas and nuclei around the lateral ventricles of the brain that are involved in the formation of emotions and memories.

Lobotomy/leucotomy: Cut through the white matter of the frontal cortex.

Magnetic resonance imaging (MRI): Technique to pick up signals that show contrasts between different tissue types (e.g. gray and white matter) by means of their characteristic resonance of protons from water.

Medial forebrain bundle (MFB): A tract of nerve fibres connecting the mesencephalon (ventral tegmental area) with the basal ganglia, the limbic system, the hypothalamus and the frontal lobe.

Mesencephalon: Midbrain. Contains the passage of the long fibre tracts from the hemispheres to the periphery and back (motor and sensory), areas for eye movement control and dopamine-releasing cells.

Minimally conscious state (MCS): Disorder of consciousness with severely impaired awareness. Patients with MCS show some directed movements, but their communication is limited to simple gestures or verbal responses. They depend on 24-hour care.

Motor cortex: Part of the frontal lobe that gives rise to the motor fibres that travel through the pyramidal or cortico-spinal tract to the anterior horn of the spinal cord.

Motor neuron disease (MND): See Amyotrophic lateral sclerosis.

Neuron: Nerve cell.

Neuroplasticity: Changes in the connectivity between neurons. These can happen at the level of an individual synapse (e.g. by changes in receptor expression or sensitivity) or by the formation or pruning of synapses.

Neurotransmitter: A chemical that mediates the communication between neurons or between neurons and muscle cells.

Obsessive compulsive disorder (OCD): Mental disorder, characterised by obsessive thoughts and compulsive actions (e.g. checking, washing, hoarding).

Opioids: A group of neurotransmitters. They are particularly important for experiences of pain and pleasure.

Organic personality disorder: A profound change in personality after a traumatic brain injury or another brain lesion. It is characterised by emotional lability, irritability, apathy, disinhibition, suspiciousness and problems with concentration and pursuit of specific goals.

Paraphilia: A group of sexual disorders characterised by "recurrent, intense sexual urges, fantasies, or behaviours that involve unusual objects, activities, or situations".[185] For a more detailed introduction to sexual disorders and their biological models see Linden, *The Biology of Psychological Disorders*.[5]

Parkinson's disease: Movement disorder characterised by the symptom triad of tremor, rigidity and slow movement initiation (hypokinesis) and by typical changes in neurons (Lewy bodies) with a loss of dopamine-producing neurons.

Periaqueductal grey matter: A collection of neurons in the brainstem. It contains opioid-sensitive neurons that are involved in the central modulation of pain.

Persistent vegetative state (PVS): Disorder of consciousness with lack of awareness. Patients do not communicate and depend on 24-hour care.

Phantom pain: Pain that develops after loss or amputation of a limb, which is located in that limb.

Positron emission tomography (PET): Imaging technique that utilises radioactive isotopes to mark specific molecules in the body.

Psychopathy: A personality disorder characterised by antisocial behaviour, lack of empathy and callousness.

Randomised controlled trial (RCT): A method to investigate the efficacy of a therapeutic intervention by comparison with appropriate control groups/ control interventions. Patients are randomly assigned to the intervention or one or several control groups. Ideally, patients and raters are "blind" to group allocation.

Schizophrenia: Mental disorder characterised by "positive" (e.g. hallucinations, delusions), "negative" (e.g. loss of enjoyment, poverty of speech) and cognitive symptoms. "Positive" does not mean that the symptoms have a positive effect but that they constitute an addition to normal perceptual and cognitive processes.

Selective serotonin reuptake inhibitors (SSRI): A group of widely prescribed antidepressants that block the uptake of the neurotransmitter serotonin into neurons and thus prolong its action.

Sexually violent predators (SVP): A term used in the law of several U.S. states. The California Welfare and Institutions Code provides the following typical definition: '"Sexually violent predator" means a person who has been convicted of a sexually violent offense against one or more victims and who has a diagnosed mental disorder that makes the person a danger to the health and safety of others in that it is likely that he or she will engage in sexually violent criminal behavior' (www.leginfo.ca.gov/cgi-bin/displaycode?section=wic&group=06001–07000&file=6600–6609.3, accessed on 13 July 2014).

Single photon emission computed tomography (SPECT): Imaging technique that utilises radioactive isotopes to mark specific molecules in the body.

Skinner box: Setup used for animal training. The standard equipment includes a lever and a source of food or drink.

Somatosensory cortex: Most anterior part of the parietal cortex that contains the neurons receiving the projections carrying tactile information from the thalamus.

Stereotactic/stereotaxic: Minimally invasive neurosurgical operation technique using insertion of instruments or electrodes with guidance by a coordinate system and a frame fixed to the skull (although frameless systems are now also available).

Subcortical: Areas below the cerebral cortex, including white matter and basal ganglia.

Substantia nigra: Part of the mesencephalon, containing dopamine-releasing neurons, which are destroyed in Parkinson's disease.

Subthalamic nucleus (STN): Part of the basal ganglia, relay station of motor signals travelling to the thalamus. Also has an associative (cognitive) and a limbic (affective) component.

Temporal lobe epilepsy (TLE): A common form of epilepsy with a focus in the temporal lobe of the brain. It is characterised by complex partial seizures, during which patients experience altered states of consciousness and engage in odd, automatic behaviours.

Thalamus: Main relay station between periphery and cortex. The main sensory input (auditory, visual and tactile modalities) travels from here to the specialised cortical areas. Also projects fibres that modulate cognitive, affective and motor processes.

Tourette's syndrome: Neuropsychiatric disorder, characterised by compulsive and often obscene utterings, tics and important comorbidities (for example with OCD).

Transcranial electrical stimulation (TES): Induction of currents in the brain through application of currents to the scalp.

Transcranial magnetic stimulation (TMS): Induction of currents in the brain through a brief application of strong magnetic fields over the skull.

Unified Parkinson's Disease Rating Scale (UPDRS): A clinical rating scale for different aspects of the severity of Parkinson's disease. It is commonly used to assess treatment effects in clinical trials.

Ventrointermedius nucleus (VIM): A structure in the thalamus and target for DBS in patients suffering from tremor.

Ventrolateral prefrontal cortex (VLPFC): Part of the frontal lobe, involved in emotion control.

Ventroposterolateral nucleus (VPL): A sensory relay nucleus of the thalamus and target for DBS in pain syndromes.

Visual cortex: Part of the cortex that receives the visual fibres from the thalamus. Located in the occipital cortex at the posterior end of the brain.

Waiting list design: A method for clinical trials in which a group receiving the intervention is compared with a group of patients on a waiting list who later to on to receive the same intervention.

White matter: Brain tissue containing mainly fibres (axon bundles).

Wolff Parkinson White (WPW) syndrome: A heart condition leading to episodes of abnormally fast heart beat.

Yale Brown Obsessive Compulsive Scale (YBOCS): A clinical rating scale for the severity of OCD symptoms that is often used to evaluate treatment outcomes.

References

1. Berger H. On the electroencephalogram of man. *Electroencephalogr Clin Neurophysiol.* 1969;Suppl 28.
2. Adrian ED, Matthews BHC. The Berger rhythm: potential changes from the occipital lobe of man. *Brain.* 1934;57(4):355–385.
3. Linden DE, Prvulovic D, Formisano E, Völlinger M, Zanella FE, Goebel R, Dierks T. The functional neuroanatomy of target detection: an fMRI study of visual and auditory oddball tasks. *Cereb Cortex.* 1999;9(8):815–823.
4. Haenschel C, Bittner RA, Waltz J, Haertling F, Wibral M, Singer W, Linden DE, Rodriguez E. Cortical oscillatory activity is critical for working memory as revealed by deficits in early-onset schizophrenia. *J Neurosci.* 2009;29(30):9481–9489.
5. Linden D. *The Biology of Psychological Disorders.* Basingstoke: Palgrave Macmillan; 2012.
6. Lee SW, Clemenson GD, Gage FH. New neurons in an aged brain. *Behav Brain Res.* 2012;227(2):497–507.
7. Doty RW, Giurgea C. Conditioned reflexes established by coupling electrical excitation of two cortical areas. In: Delafresneye JF, ed. *Brain Mechanisms and Learning.* Oxford: Oxford University Press.
8. Jackson A, Mavoori J, Fetz EE. Long-term motor cortex plasticity induced by an electronic neural implant. *Nature.* 2006;444(7115):56–60.
9. Hebb DO. *The Organization of Behaviour: A Neuropsychological Theory.* [S.l.]: Chapman and Hall; 1949.
10. Olds J, Olds ME. Interference and learning in palaeocortical systems. In: Delafresneye JF, ed. *Brain Mechanisms and Learning.* Oxford: Oxford University Press; 1961:153–187.
11. Fetz EE. Operant conditioning of cortical unit activity. *Science.* 1969;163(3870):955–958.
12. Koralek AC, Jin X, Long JD, Costa RM, Carmena JM. Corticostriatal plasticity is necessary for learning intentional neuroprosthetic skills. *Nature.* 2012;483(7389):331–335.
13. Hilgard ER, Marquis DG. *Hilgard and Marquis' Conditioning and Learning.* 2nd ed. New York: Appleton-Century-Crofts; 1961.
14. Rescorla RA, Solomon RL. Two-process learning theory: relationships between Pavlovian conditioning and instrumental learning. *Psychol Rev.* 1967;74(3):151–182.
15. Miller NE. Learning of visceral and glandular responses. *Science.* 1969;163(3866):434–445.
16. Birbaumer N, Cohen L. Brain-computer interfaces: communication and restoration of movement in paralysis. *J Physiol.* 2007;579(3):621–636.
17. Wolpaw JR, Birbaumer N, McFarland DJ, Pfurtscheller G, Vaughan TM. Brain-computer interfaces for communication and control. *Clin Neurophysiol.* 2002;113(6):767–791.

18. Kaufmann T, Völker S, Gunesch L, Kübler A. Spelling is just a click away – a user-centered brain-computer interface including auto-calibration and predictive text entry. *Front Neurosci.* 2012;6:72.

19. Birbaumer N, Ghanayim N, Hinterberger T, Iversen I, Kotchoubey B, Kübler A, Perelmouter J, Taub E, Flor H. A spelling device for the paralysed. *Nature.* 1999;398(6725):297–298.

20. Kübler A, Holz E, Botrel L. Addendum. *Brain.* 2013;136(6):2005–2006.

21. De Massari D, Ruf CA, Furdea A, Matuz T, van der Heiden L, Halder S, Silvoni S, Birbaumer N. Brain communication in the locked-in state. *Brain.* 2013;136(6):1989–2000.

22. Linden DE. The challenges and promise of neuroimaging in psychiatry. *Neuron.* 2012;73(1):8–22.

23. Dierks T, Linden DE, Jandl M, Formisano E, Goebel R, Lanfermann H, Singer W. Activation of Heschl's gyrus during auditory hallucinations. *Neuron.* 1999;22(3):615–621.

24. Linden DE, Thornton K, Kuswanto CN, Johnston SJ, van de Ven V, Jackson MC. The brain's voices: comparing nonclinical auditory hallucinations and imagery. *Cereb Cortex.* 2011;21(2):330–337.

25. Michelon P, Vettel JM, Zacks JM. Lateral somatotopic organization during imagined and prepared movements. *J Neurophysiol.* 2006;95(2):811–822.

26. Sorger B, Reithler J, Dahmen B, Goebel R. a real-time fMRI-based spelling device immediately enabling robust motor-independent communication. *Curr Biol.* 2012;22(14):1333–1338.

27. Sorger B, Dahmen B, Reithler J, Gosseries O, Maudoux A, Laureys S, Goebel R. Another kind of "BOLD Response": answering multiple-choice questions via online decoded single-trial brain signals. *Prog Brain Res.* 2009;177:275–292.

28. Monti M, Vanhaudenhuyse A, Coleman M, Boly M, Pickard JD, Tshibanda L, Owen AM, Laureys S. Willful modulation of brain activity in disorders of consciousness. *N Engl J Med.* 2010;362(7):579–589.

29. Richmond S, Rees G, Edwards SJL. *I Know What You're Thinking: Brain Imaging and Mental Privacy.* Oxford: Oxford University Press; 2012.

30. Jackson A, Fetz EE. Interfacing with the computational brain. *IEEE Trans Neural Syst Rehabil Eng.* 2011;19(5):534–541.

31. Velliste M, Perel S, Spalding MC, Whitford AS, Schwartz AB. Cortical control of a prosthetic arm for self-feeding. *Nature.* 2008;453(7198):1098–1101.

32. Buch E, Weber C, Cohen LG, Braun C, Dimyan MA, Ard T, Mellinger J, Caria A, Soekadar S, Fourkas A, Birbaumer N. Think to move: a neuro-magnetic brain-computer interface (BCI) system for chronic stroke. *Stroke.* 2008;39(3):910–917.

33. O'Doherty JE, Lebedev MA, Ifft PJ, Zhuang KZ, Shokur S, Bleuler H, Nicolelis MA. Active tactile exploration using a brain-machine-brain interface. *Nature.* 2011;479(7372):228–231.

34. Moritz CT, Perlmutter SI, Fetz EE. Direct control of paralysed muscles by cortical neurons. *Nature.* 2008;456(7222):639–642.

35. Ethier C, Oby ER, Bauman MJ, Miller LE. Restoration of grasp following paralysis through brain-controlled stimulation of muscles. *Nature.* 2012;485(7398):368–371.

36. Rothschild RM. Neuroengineering tools/applications for bidirectional inter-faces, brain-computer interfaces, and neuroprosthetic implants – a review of recent progress. *Front Neuroeng.* 2010;3:112.
37. Hochberg LR, Serruya MD, Friehs GM, Mukand JA, Saleh M, Caplan AH, Branner A, Chen D, Penn RD, Donoghue JP. Neuronal ensemble control of prosthetic devices by a human with tetraplegia. *Nature.* 2006;442(7099):164–171.
38. Hochberg LR, Bacher D, Jarosiewicz B, Masse NY, Simeral JD, Vogel J, Haddadin S, Liu J, Cash SS, van der Smagt P, Donoghue JP. Reach and grasp by people with tetraplegia using a neurally controlled robotic arm. *Nature.* 2012;485(7398):372–375.
39. Lucretius Carus T, Rouse WHD, Smith MF. *De rerum natura.* Cambridge, Mass.: Harvard University Press; 1975.
40. Kandel ER. Biology and the future of psychoanalysis: a new intellectual framework for psychiatry revisited. *Am J Psychiatry.* 1999;156(4):505–524.
41. Penfield W. Conditioning the uncommitted cortex for language learning. *Brain.* 1965;88(4):787–798.
42. Penfield W, Perot P. The brain's record of auditory and visual experience. A final summary and discussion. *Brain.* 1963;86(4):595–696.
43. Ramey ER, O'Doherty DS. *Electrical Studies on the Unanesthetized Brain; a Symposium with 49 Participants.* New York: P. B. Hoeber; 1960.
44. Valenstein ES. *Brain control. A Critical Examination of Brain Stimulation and Psychosurgery.* New York: John Wiley & Sons; 1973.
45. Eibl-Eibesfeldt I. Technik der Vergleichenden Verhaltensforschung. In: Helmcke J, von Lengerken H, Starck D, eds. *Handbuch der Zoologie.* 1962;10(2):19–21.
46. Delgado JMR. *Physical Control of the Mind; toward a Psychocivilized Society.* 1st ed. New York: Harper & Row; 1969.
47. Heath RG. *Exploring the Mind-Brain Relationship.* Baton Rouge: Moran Printing, Inc.; 1996.
48. Olds J. Self-stimulation of the brain; its use to study local effects of hunger, sex, and drugs. *Science.* 1958;127(3294):315–324.
49. Olds J. Hypothalamic substrates of reward. *Physiol Rev.* 1962;42:554–604.
50. Olds J. Self-stimulation experiments. *Science.* 1963;140(3563):218–220.
51. Porter RW, Conrad DG, Brady JV. Some neural and behavioral corre-lates of electrical self-stimulation of the limbic system. *J Exp Anal Behav.* 1959;2(1):43–55.
52. Singh J, Desiraju T, Raju TR. Comparison of intracranial self-stimulation evoked from lateral hypothalamus and ventral tegmentum: analysis based on stimulation parameters and behavioural response characteristics. *Brain Res Bull.* 1996;41(6):399–408.
53. Ahmed SH. The science of making drug-addicted animals. *Neuroscience.* 2012;211:107–125.
54. Wise RA. Addictive drugs and brain stimulation reward. *Annu Rev Neurosci.* 1996;19:319–340.
55. Gallistel CR, Karras D. Pimozide and amphetamine have opposing effects on the reward summation function. *Pharmacol Biochem Behav.* 1984;20(1):73–77.
56. Hoebel BG, Monaco AP, Hernandez L, Aulisi EF, Stanley BG, Lenard L. Self-injection of amphetamine directly into the brain. *Psychopharmacology (Berl).* 1983;81(2):158–163.

57. Heath RG, Mickle WA. Evaluation of seven years' experience with depth electrode studies in human patients. In: Ramey ER, O'Doherty DS, eds. *Electrical Studies on the Unanaesthetized Brain*. New York: Hoeber; 1960.

58. Bergman H, Wichmann T, DeLong MR. Reversal of experimental parkinsonism by lesions of the subthalamic nucleus. *Science*. 1990;249(4975):1436–1438.

59. Kringelbach ML, Jenkinson N, Owen SL, Aziz TZ. Translational principles of deep brain stimulation. *Nat Rev Neurosci*. 2007;8(8):623–635.

60. Okun MS. Deep-brain stimulation for Parkinson's disease. *N Engl J Med*. 2012;367(16):1529–1538.

61. Kumar R, Lozano AM, Kim YJ, Hutchison WD, Sime E, Halket E, Lang AE. Double-blind evaluation of subthalamic nucleus deep brain stimulation in advanced Parkinson's disease. *Neurology*. 1998;51(3):850–855.

62. Kumar R, Lozano AM, Sime E, Halket E, Lang AE. Comparative effects of unilateral and bilateral subthalamic nucleus deep brain stimulation. *Neurology*. 1999;53(3):561–566.

63. Johnson MD, Miocinovic S, McIntyre CC, Vitek JL. Mechanisms and targets of deep brain stimulation in movement disorders. *Neurotherapeutics*. 2008;5(2):294–308.

64. Rosa M, Giannicola G, Marceglia S, Fumagalli M, Barbieri S, Priori A. Neurophysiology of deep brain stimulation. *Int Rev Neurobiol*. 2012;107:23–55.

65. Albanese A, Romito L. Deep brain stimulation for Parkinson's disease: where do we stand? *Front Neurol*. 2011;2:33.

66. Schuepbach WM, Rau J, Knudsen K, Volkmann J, Krack P, Timmermann L, Hälbig TD, Hesekamp H, Navarro SM, Meier N, Falk D, Mehdorn M, Paschen S, Maarouf M, Barbe MT, Fink GR, Kupsch A, Gruber D, Schneider GH, Seigneuret E, Kistner A, Chaynes P, Ory-Magne F, Brefel Courbon C, Vesper J, Schnitzler A, Wojtecki L, Houeto JL, Bataille B, Maltête D, Damier P, Raoul S, Sixel-Doering F, Hellwig D, Gharabaghi A, Krüger R, Pinsker MO, Amtage F, Régis JM, Witjas T, Thobois S, Mertens P, Kloss M, Hartmann A, Oertel WH, Post B, Speelman H, Agid Y, Schade-Brittinger C, Deuschl G; EARLYSTIM Study Group. Neurostimulation for Parkinson's disease with early motor complications. *N Engl J Med*. 2013;368(7):610–622.

67. Deuschl G, Raethjen J, Hellriegel H, Elble R. Treatment of patients with essential tremor. *Lancet Neurol*. 2011;10(2):148–161.

68. Collins KL, Lehmann EM, Patil PG. Deep brain stimulation for movement disorders. *Neurobiol Dis*. 2010;38(3):338–345.

69. Nizard J, Raoul S, Nguyen JP, Lefaucheur JP. Invasive stimulation therapies for the treatment of refractory pain. *Discov Med*. 2012;14(77):237–246.

70. Goethals I, Jacobs F, Van der Linden C, Caemaert J, Audenaert K. Brain activation associated with deep brain stimulation causing dissociation in a patient with Tourette's syndrome. *J Trauma Dissociation*. 2008;9(4):543–549.

71. Miocinovic S, Somayajula S, Chitnis S, Vitek JL. History, applications, and mechanisms of deep brain stimulation. *JAMA Neurol*. 2013;70(2):163–171.

72. Rodriguez-Oroz MC, Jahanshahi M, Krack P, Litvan I, Macias R, Bezard E, Obeso JA. Initial clinical manifestations of Parkinson's disease: features and pathophysiological mechanisms. *Lancet Neurol*. 2009;8(12):1128–1139.

73. Obeso JA, Rodríguez-Oroz MC, Benitez-Temino B, Blesa FJ, Guridi J, Marin C, Rodriguez M. Functional organization of the basal ganglia: therapeutic implications for Parkinson's disease. *Mov Disord*. 2008;23 Suppl 3:S548–559.

74. Mallet L, Schüpbach M, N'Diaye K, Remy P, Bardinet E, Czernecki V, Welter ML, Pelissolo A, Ruberg M, Agid Y, Yelnik J. Stimulation of subterritories of the subthalamic nucleus reveals its role in the integration of the emotional and motor aspects of behavior. *Proc Natl Acad Sci U S A.* 2007;104(25):10661–10666.

75. Massano J, Garrett C. Deep brain stimulation and cognitive decline in Parkinson's disease: a clinical review. *Front Neurol.* 2012;3:66.

76. Ardouin C, Voon V, Worbe Y, Abouazar N, Czernecki V, Hosseini H, Pelissolo A, Moro E, Lhommée E, Lang AE, Agid Y, Benabid AL, Pollak P, Mallet L, Krack P. Pathological gambling in Parkinson's disease improves on chronic subthalamic nucleus stimulation. *Mov Disord.* 2006;21(11):1941–1946.

77. Lhommée E, Klinger H, Thobois S, Schmitt E, Ardouin C, Bichon A, Kistner A, Fraix V, Xie J, Aya Kombo M, Chabardès S, Seigneuret E, Benabid AL, Mertens P, Polo G, Carnicella S, Quesada JL, Bosson JL, Broussolle E, Pollak P, Krack P. Subthalamic stimulation in Parkinson's disease: restoring the balance of motivated behaviours. *Brain.* 2012;135(5):1463–1477.

78. Gazzaniga MS. *Who's in Charge?: Free Will and the Science of the Brain.* 1st ed. New York, NY: HarperCollins; 2011.

79. Berrios GE. The origins of psychosurgery: Shaw, Burckhardt and Moniz. *Hist Psychiatry.* 1997;8(29):61–81.

80. Pressman JD. *Last Resort: Psychosurgery and the Limits of Medicine.* Cambridge: Cambridge University Press; 1998.

81. El-Hai J. *The Lobotomist: A Maverick Medical Genius and His Tragic Quest to Rid the World of Mental Illness.* Hoboken, N.J.: J. Wiley; 2005.

82. Freeman WJ, Watts JW. *Psychosurgery. On the Treatment of Mental Disorders and Intractable Pain.* 2nd ed. Blackwell Scientific Publications: Oxford; Fort Worth; 1950: xxviii, 598

83. Freeman W. Transorbital lobotomy. *Am J Psychiatry.* 1949;105(10):734–740.

84. Kalinowsky LB, Hoch PH. *Somatic Treatments in Psychiatry; Pharmacotherapy; Convulsive, Insulin, Surgical, Other Methods.* New York: Grune & Stratton; 1961.

85. O'Callaghan MAJ, Carroll D. *Psychosurgery: A Scientific Analysis.* Lancaster: MTP Press; 1982.

86. Rees WL, Jones AM. An evaluation of the Rorschach test as a prognostic aid in the treatment of schizophrenia by insulin coma therapy, electronarcosis, electroconvulsive therapy and leucotomy. *J Ment Sci.* 1951;97(409):681–689.

87. Shorter E, Healy D. *Shock Therapy. The History of Electroconvulsive Treatment in Mental Illness.* New Brunswick, NJ: Rutgers University Press; 2007.

88. Narabayashi H, Nagao T, Saito Y, Yoshida M, Nagahata M. Stereotaxic amygdalotomy for behavior disorders. *Arch Neurol.* 1963;9(1):1–16.

89. Sano K, Yoshioka M, Ogashiwa M, Ishijima B, Ohye C. Postero-medial hypothalamotomy in the treatment of aggressive behaviors. *Confin Neurol.* 1966;27(1):164–167.

90. Lee GP, Bechara A, Adolphs R, Arena J, Meador KJ, Loring DW, Smith JR. Clinical and physiological effects of stereotaxic bilateral amygdalotomy for intractable aggression. *J Neuropsychiatry Clin Neurosci.* 1998;10(4):413–420.

91. Müller D. Psychiatrische Chirurgie. In: Arnold H, ed. *Neurochirurgie in Deutschland: Geschichte und Gegenwart. 50 Jahre Deutsche Gesellschaft für Neurochirurgie.* Boston: Blackwell; 2001:258–266.

92. Timmann H-D, Müller D. *Stereotaktische Hirnoperationen bei sexuell Devianten. Darstellung und Interpretation der Ergebnisse einer katamnestischen Untersuchung.* Hamburg; 2003.
93. Dieckmann G, Schneider-Jonietz B, Schneider H. Psychiatric and neuropsychological findings after stereotactic hypothalamotomy, in cases of extreme sexual aggressivity. *Acta Neurochir Suppl (Wien).* 1988;44:163–166.
94. Greenberg B, Rauch S, Haber S. Invasive circuitry-based neurotherapeutics: stereotactic ablation and deep brain stimulation for OCD. *Neuropsychopharmacology.* 2010;35(1):317–336.
95. Ballantine HT, Bouckoms AJ, Thomas EK, Giriunas IE. Treatment of psychiatric illness by stereotactic cingulotomy. *Biol Psychiatry.* 1987;22(7):807–819.
96. Sheth SA, Neal J, Tangherlini F, Mian MK, Gentil A, Cosgrove GR, Eskandar EN, Dougherty DD. Limbic system surgery for treatment-refractory obsessive-compulsive disorder: a prospective long-term follow-up of 64 patients. *J Neurosurg.* 2013;118(3):491–497.
97. Christmas D, Eljamel MS, Butler S, Hazari H, MacVicar R, Steele JD, Livingstone A, Matthews K. Long term outcome of thermal anterior capsulotomy for chronic, treatment refractory depression. *J Neurol Neurosurg Psychiatry.* 2011;82(6):594–600.
98. Sachdev PS, Sachdev J. Long-term outcome of neurosurgery for the treatment of resistant depression. *J Neuropsychiatry Clin Neurosci.* 2005;17(4):478–485.
99. Partridge MW. *Pre-Frontal Leucotomy. A Survey of 300 Cases Personally Followed Over 1 1/2–3 Years.* Oxford: Blackwell Scientific Publications; 1950.
100. Cosgrove GR. Cingulotomy for depression and OCD. In: Lozano AM, Gildenberg PL, Tasker RR, eds. *Textbook of Stereotactic and Functional Neurosurgery.* 2nd ed. Berlin: Springer; 2009:2887–2896.
101. Medvedev SV, Anichkov AD, Poliakov II. [Physiological mechanisms of the effectiveness of bilateral stereotactic cingulotomy in treatment of strong psychological dependence in drug addiction]. *Fiziol Cheloveka.* 2003;29(4):117–123.
102. Orellana C. Controversy over brain surgery for heroin addiction in Russia. *Lancet Neurol.* 2002;1(6):333.
103. Peciña S, Smith K, Berridge K. Hedonic hot spots in the brain. *Neuroscientist.* 2006;12(6):500–511.
104. Münte TF, Heinze HJ, Visser-Vandewalle V. Deep brain stimulation as a therapy for alcohol addiction. *Curr Top Behav Neurosci.* 2013;13:709–727.
105. Sun B, Zhan S, Li D, Wu H. Surgical Treatment for Refractory Addictions. In: Krames ES, Peckham PH, Rezai AR, eds. *Neuromodulation.* Amsterdam: Academic Press; 2009.
106. Ge S, Chang C, Adler JR, Zhao H, Chang X, Gao L, Wu H, Wang J, Li N, Wang X, Gao G. Long-term changes in the personality and psychopathological profile of opiate addicts after nucleus accumbens ablative surgery are associated with treatment outcome. *Stereotact Funct Neurosurg.* 2013;91(1):30–44.
107. Mallet L, Polosan M, Jaafari N, Baup N, Welter ML, Fontaine D, du Montcel ST, Yelnik J, Chéreau I, Arbus C, Raoul S, Aouizerate B, Damier P, Chabardès S, Czernecki V, Ardouin C, Krebs MO, Bardinet E, Chaynes P, Burbaud P, Cornu P, Derost P, Bougerol T, Bataille B, Mattei V, Dormont D, Devaux B, Vérin M, Houeto JL, Pollak P, Benabid AL, Agid Y, Krack P, Millet B, Pelissolo

A; STOC Study Group. Subthalamic nucleus stimulation in severe obsessive-compulsive disorder. *N Engl J Med.* 2008;359(20):2121–2134.
108. Piedad JC, Rickards HE, Cavanna AE. What patients with gilles de la tourette syndrome should be treated with deep brain stimulation and what is the best target? *Neurosurgery.* 2012;71(1):173–192.
109. Goodman WK, Alterman RL. Deep brain stimulation for intractable psychiatric disorders. *Annu Rev Med.* 2012;63:511–524.
110. Bewernick BH, Kayser S, Sturm V, Schlaepfer TE. Long-term effects of nucleus accumbens deep brain stimulation in treatment-resistant depression: evidence for sustained efficacy. *Neuropsychopharmacology.* 2012;37(9):1975–1985.
111. Holtzheimer PE, Kelley ME, Gross RE, Filkowski MM, Garlow SJ, Barrocas A, Wint D, Craighead MC, Kozarsky J, Chismar R, Moreines JL, Mewes K, Posse PR, Gutman DA, Mayberg HS. Subcallosal cingulate deep brain stimulation for treatment-resistant unipolar and bipolar depression. *Arch Gen Psychiatry.* 2012;69(2):150–158.
112. Lozano A, Mayberg H, Giacobbe P, Hamani C, Craddock R, Kennedy S. Subcallosal cingulate gyrus deep brain stimulation for treatment-resistant depression. *Biol Psychiatry.* 2008;64(6):461–467.
113. Lozano AM, Lipsman N. Probing and regulating dysfunctional circuits using deep brain stimulation. *Neuron.* 2013;77(3):406–424.
114. Schlaepfer TE, Bewernick BH, Kayser S, Mädler B, Coenen VA. Rapid effects of deep brain stimulation for treatment-resistant major depression. *Biol Psychiatry.* 2013;73(12):1204–1212.
115. Höflich A, Savli M, Comasco E, Moser U, Novak K, Kasper S, Lanzenberger R. Neuropsychiatric deep brain stimulation for translational neuroimaging. *Neuroimage.* 2013;79:30–41.
116. Kuhn J, Möller M, Treppmann JF, Bartsch C, Lenartz D, Gruendler TO, Maarouf M, Brosig A, Barnikol UB, Klosterkötter J, Sturm V. Deep brain stimulation of the nucleus accumbens and its usefulness in severe opioid addiction. *Mol Psychiatry.* 2014;19(2):145–6.
117. Luigjes J, van den Brink W, Feenstra M, van den Munckhof P, Schuurman PR, Schippers R, Mazaheri A, De Vries TJ, Denys D. Deep brain stimulation in addiction: a review of potential brain targets. *Mol Psychiatry.* 2012;17(6):572–583.
118. Carter A, Bell E, Racine E, Hall W. Ethical issues raised by proposals to treat addiction using deep brain stimulation. *Neuroethics.* 2011;4(2):129–142.
119. Lipsman N, Woodside DB, Giacobbe P, Hamani C, Carter JC, Norwood SJ, Sutandar K, Staab R, Elias G, Lyman CH, Smith GS, Lozano AM. Subcallosal cingulate deep brain stimulation for treatment-refractory anorexia nervosa: a phase 1 pilot trial. *Lancet.* 2013;381(9875):1361–1370.
120. Krames E, Peckham PH, Rezai AR. *Neuromodulation.* London: Academic; 2009.
121. Hariz MI, Hariz GM. Hyping deep brain stimulation in psychiatry could lead to its demise. *BMJ.* 2012;345:e5447.
122. Miller NE. *Biofeedback and Self-Control, 1973: An Aldine Annual on the Regulation of Bodily Processes and Consciousness.* Chicago: Aldine; 1974.
123. Sterman MB. The Role of Sensorimotor Rhythmic EEG Activity in the Etiology and Treatment of Generalized Motor Seizures. In: Elbert T,

Rockstroh B, Lutzenberger W, Birbaumer N, eds. *Self-Regulation of the Brain and Behavior.* Berlin: Springer; 1984:95–106.

124. Lubar JF. Applications of Operant Conditioning of the EEG for the Management of Epileptic Seizures. In: Elbert T, Rockstroh B, Lutzenberger W, Birbaumer N, eds. *Self-Regulation of the Brain and Behavior.* Berlin: Springer; 1984:107–136.

125. Stamm JS. Performance enhancements with cortical negative slow potential shifts in monkey and human. In: Elbert T, Rockstroh B, Lutzenberger W, Birbaumer N, eds. *Self-Regulation of the Brain and Behavior.* Berlin: Springer; 1984:199–215.

126. Bauer H. Regulation of slow brain potentials affects task performance. In: Elbert T, Rockstroh B, Lutzenberger W, Birbaumer N, eds. *Self-Regulation of the Brain and Behavior.* Berlin: Springer; 1984:216–226.

127. Gruzelier J, Egner T, Vernon D. Validating the efficacy of neurofeedback for optimising performance. *Prog Brain Res.* 2006;159:421–431.

128. Powell DH. Treating individuals with debilitating performance anxiety: an introduction. *J Clin Psychol.* 2004;60(8):801–808.

129. Raymond J, Sajid I, Parkinson LA, Gruzelier JH. Biofeedback and dance performance: a preliminary investigation. *Appl Psychophysiol Biofeedback.* 2005;30(1):64–73.

130. Ros T, Moseley MJ, Bloom PA, Benjamin L, Parkinson LA, Gruzelier JH. Optimizing microsurgical skills with EEG neurofeedback. *BMC Neurosci.* 2009;10:87.

131. Gevensleben H, Holl B, Albrecht B, Vogel C, Schlamp D, Kratz O, Studer P, Rothenberger A, Moll GH, Heinrich H. Is neurofeedback an efficacious treatment for ADHD? A randomised controlled clinical trial. *J Child Psychol Psychiatry.* 2009;50(7):780–789.

132. Gevensleben H, Holl B, Albrecht B, Schlamp D, Kratz O, Studer P, Rothenberger A, Moll GH, Heinrich H. Neurofeedback training in children with ADHD: 6-month follow-up of a randomised controlled trial. *Eur Child Adolesc Psychiatry.* 2010;19(9):715–724.

133. Gevensleben H, Rothenberger A, Moll GH, Heinrich H. Neurofeedback in children with ADHD: validation and challenges. *Expert Rev Neurother.* 2012;12(4):447–460.

134. Lofthouse N, Arnold LE, Hersch S, Hurt E, Debeus R. A review of neurofeedback treatment for pediatric ADHD. *J Atten Disord.* 2012;16(5):351–372.

135. Sonuga-Barke EJ, Brandeis D, Cortese S, Daley D, Ferrin M, Holtmann M, Stevenson J, Danckaerts M, van der Oord S, Döpfner M, Dittmann RW, Simonoff E, Zuddas A, Banaschewski T, Buitelaar J, Coghill D, Hollis C, Konofal E, Lecendreux M, Wong IC, Sergeant J; European ADHD Guidelines Group. Nonpharmacological interventions for ADHD: systematic review and meta-analyses of randomized controlled trials of dietary and psychological treatments. *Am J Psychiatry.* 2013;170(3):275–289.

136. (NICE) NIfCE. *Attention Deficit Hyperactivity Disorder. The NICE Guideline on Diagnosis and Management of ADHD in children, young people and adults.* London: The British Psychological Society and The Royal College of Psychiatrists; 2009.

137. Jager S, Muller KW, Ruckes C, Wittig T, Batra A, Musalek M, Mann K, Wölfling K, Beutel ME. Effects of a manualized short-term treatment of

internet and computer game addiction (STICA): study protocol for a randomized controlled trial. *Trials*. 2012;13(1):43.

138. deCharms R, Maeda F, Glover G, Ludlow D, Pauly JM, Soneji D, Gabrieli JD, Mackey SC. Control over brain activation and pain learned by using real-time functional MRI. *Proc Natl Acad Sci U S A*. 2005;102(51):18626–18631.

139. Bandura A. Social cognitive theory: an agentic perspective. *Asian Journal of Social Psychology*. 1999;2(1):21–41.

140. Subramanian L, Hindle JV, Johnston S, Roberts MV, Husain M, Goebel R, Linden D. Real-time functional magnetic resonance imaging neurofeedback for treatment of Parkinson's disease. *J Neurosci*. 2011;31(45):16309–16317.

141. Linden DE, Habes I, Johnston SJ, Linden S, Tatineni R, Subramanian L, Sorger B, Healy D, Goebel R. Real-time self-regulation of emotion networks in patients with depression. *PLoS One*. 2012;7(6):e38115.

142. Hawkinson JE, Ross AJ, Parthasarathy S, Scott DJ, Laramee EA, Posecion LJ, Rekshan WR, Sheau KE, Njaka ND, Bayley PJ, deCharms RC. Quantification of adverse events associated with functional MRI Scanning and with real-time fMRI-based training. *Int J Behav Med*. 2012;19(3):372–381.

143. Esmail S, Linden D. Emotion regulation networks and neurofeedback in depression. *Cognitive Sciences*. 2011;6(2).

144. Nachev P, Kennard C, Husain M. Functional role of the supplementary and pre-supplementary motor areas. *Nat Rev Neurosci*. 2008;9(11):856–869.

145. de la Fuente-Fernández R, Ruth TJ, Sossi V, Schulzer M, Calne DB, Stoessl AJ. Expectation and dopamine release: mechanism of the placebo effect in Parkinson's disease. *Science*. 2001;293(5532):1164–1166.

146. Little S, Pogosyan A, Neal S, Zavala B, Zrinzo L, Hariz M, Foltynie T, Limousin P, Ashkan K, FitzGerald J, Green AL, Aziz TZ, Brown P. Adaptive deep brain stimulation in advanced Parkinson disease. *Ann Neurol*. 2013;74(3):449–457.

147. Kim MC, Lee TK. Stereotactic lesioning for mental illness. *Acta Neurochir Suppl*. 2008;101:39–43.

148. Dotchin C, Walker R. The management of Parkinson's disease in sub-Saharan Africa. *Expert Rev Neurother*. 2012;12(6):661–666.

149. Williams A, Gill S, Varma T, Jenkinson C, Quinn N, Mitchell R, Scott R, Ives N, Rick C, Daniels J, Patel S, Wheatley K; PD SURG Collaborative Group. Deep brain stimulation plus best medical therapy versus best medical therapy alone for advanced Parkinson's disease (PD SURG trial): a randomised, open-label trial. *Lancet Neurol*. 2010;9(6):581–591.

150. Merola A, Rizzi L, Zibetti M, Artusi CA, Montanaro E, Angrisano S, Lanotte M, Rizzone MG, Lopiano L. Medical therapy and subthalamic deep brain stimulation in advanced Parkinson's disease: a different long-term outcome? *J Neurol Neurosurg Psychiatry*. 2014;85(5):552–559.

151. Langevin JP, De Salles AA, Kosoyan HP, Krahl SE. Deep brain stimulation of the amygdala alleviates post-traumatic stress disorder symptoms in a rat model. *J Psychiatr Res*. 2010;44(16):1241–1245.

152. Taghva A, Oluigbo C, Corrigan J, Rezai AR. Posttraumatic stress disorder: neurocircuitry and implications for potential deep brain stimulation. *Stereotact Funct Neurosurg*. 2013;91(4):207–219.

153. Torres CV, Sola RG, Pastor J, Pedrosa M, Navas M, García-Navarrete E, Ezquiaga E, García-Camba E. Long-term results of posteromedial hypothalamic deep

brain stimulation for patients with resistant aggressiveness. *J Neurosurg.* 2013;119(2):277–287.

154. Broggi G, Franzini A. Treatment of Aggressive Behavior. In: Lozano AM, Gildenberg PL, Tasker RR, eds. *Textbook of Stereotactic and Functional Neurosurgery.* 2nd ed. Berlin: Springer; 2009:2971–2977.

155. Sargant WW, Hill D, Slater E. *An Introduction to Physical Methods of Treatment in Psychiatry.* 3rd ed. Edinburgh; London: E. & S. Livingstone; 1954.

156. Valenstein ES, ed. *The Psychosurgery Debate.* San Francisco: W H Freeman; 1980.

157. Doshi PK. Surgical treatment of obsessive compulsive disorders: Current status. *Indian J Psychiatry.* 2009;51(3):216–221.

158. Scoville W. Psychosurgery and other lesions of the brain affecting human behaviour. In: Hitchcock ER, ed. *Psychosurgery.* Springfield, Ill.: C C Thomas; 1972.

159. Synofzik M, Schlaepfer TE. Electrodes in the brain – ethical criteria for research and treatment with deep brain stimulation for neuropsychiatric disorders. *Brain Stimul.* 2011;4(1):7–16.

160. Synofzik M, Fins JJ, Schlaepfer TE. A neuromodulation experience registry for deep brain stimulation studies in psychiatric research: rationale and recommendations for implementation. *Brain Stimul.* 2012;5(4):653–655.

161. Diemath HE, Nievoll A. [Stereotaxic intervention in the amygdaloid nucleus and in the opposite dorso-median nucleus in erethismic children]. *Confin Neurol.* 1966;27(1):172–180.

162. Fountas KN, Smith JR. Historical evolution of stereotactic amygdalotomy for the management of severe aggression. *J Neurosurg.* 2007;106(4):710–713.

163. Chavkin S. *The Mind Stealers: Psychosurgery and Mind Control.* Boston: Houghton Mifflin; 1978.

164. *Mental Disability Law Reporter.* 1976–1977.

165. Blatte H. State prisons and the use of behavior control. *Hastings Cent Rep.* 1974;4(4):11.

166. Mark VH, Ervin FR. *Violence and the Brain.* 1st ed. New York: Medical Dept.; 1970.

167. Lichterman BL. On the history of psychosurgery in Russia. *Acta Neurochir (Wien).* 1993;125(1–4):1–4.

168. Lane C. *Shyness: How Normal Behavior Became a Sickness.* New Haven, Conn.; London: Yale University Press; 2007.

169. Healy D. *Images of Trauma: From Hysteria to Post-Traumatic Stress Disorder.* London: Faber; 1993.

170. Shorter E. *A History of Psychiatry: From the Era of the Asylum to the Age of Prozac.* New York: John Wiley & Sons; 1997.

171. Knight G. Further observations from an experience of 660 cases of stereotactic tractotomy. *Postgrad Med J.* 1973;49(578):845–854.

172. Kleinig J. *Ethical Issues in Psychosurgery.* London; Boston: Allen & Unwin; 1985.

173. Dennis JA, Khan O, Ferriter M, Huband N, Powney MJ, Duggan C. Psychological interventions for adults who have sexually offended or are at risk of offending. *Cochrane Database Syst Rev.* 2012;12:CD007507.

174. Eher R, Pfäfflin F. Adult sexual offender treatment – is it effective? In: Boer D, ed. *International Perspectives on the Assessment and Treatment of*

Sexual Offenders: Theory, Practice, and Research. Oxford: Wiley-Blackwell; 2011:3–12.

175. Janus ES. Preventive detention of sex offenders: the American experience versus international human rights norms. *Behav Sci Law.* 2013;31(3):328–343.

176. McSherry B, Keyzer P. *Sex Offenders and Preventive Detention: Politics, Policy and Practice.* Annandale, N.S.W.: Federation Press; 2009.

177. Merkel R. *Intervening in the Brain: Changing Psyche and Society.* Berlin: Springer; 2007.

178. Racine E, Waldman S, Palmour N, Risse D, Illes J. "Currents of hope": neurostimulation techniques in U.S. and U.K. print media. *Camb Q Healthc Ethics.* 2007;16(3):312–316.

179. Lozano AM, Gildenberg PL, Tasker RR, eds. *Textbook of Stereotactic and Functional Neurosurgery.* 2nd ed. Berlin: Springer; 2009.

180. Fins JJ, Mayberg HS, Nuttin B, Kubu CS, Galert T, Sturm V, Stoppenbrink K, Merkel R, Schlaepfer TE. Misuse of the FDA's humanitarian device exemption in deep brain stimulation for obsessive-compulsive disorder. *Health Aff (Millwood).* 2011;30(2):302–311.

181. Appleby BS, Rabins PV. Ethical considerations in psychiatric surgery. In: Lozano AM, Gildenberg PL, Tasker RR, eds. *Textbook of Stereotactic and Functional Neurosurgery.* 2nd ed. Berlin: Springer; 2009:2855–2866.

182. Schiff ND. Disorders of consciousness. In: Lozano A, ed. *Stereotactic and Functional Neurosurgery.* Berlin: Springer; 2009:2981–2990.

183. Fins J. Deep brain stimulation: ethical issues in clinical practice and neurosurgical research. In: Krames ES, Peckham PH, Rezai AR, eds. *Neuromodulation.* Amsterdam: Academic Press; 2009.

184. Glannon W. Neuromodulation, Agency and Autonomy. *Brain Topogr.* 2014; 27(1):46–54.

185. *Diagnostic and Statistical Manual of Mental Disorders: DSM-IV-TR.* 4th ed., text revision. Washington, DC: American Psychiatric Association; 2000.

Index